REFERENCE

D1216208

WITHDRAWN

REFERENCE

Oxford Handbook of
Nurse
Prescribing

Sue Beckwith

Doctoral Research Fellow with
the Consortium for Healthcare Research,
Centre of Research in Primary and Community Care
(CRIPACC), University of Hertfordshire, UK

and

Penny Franklin

Senior Lecturer/Programme Lead,
Non-medical Prescribing,
University of Plymouth, UK

and

Non-medical Prescribing Development Lead,

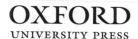

OXFORD
UNIVERSITY PRESS

BP 45

OXFORD
UNIVERSITY PRESS

Great Clarendon Street, Oxford OX2 6DP

Oxford University Press is a department of the University of Oxford.
It furthers the University's objective of excellence in research, scholarship,
and education by publishing worldwide in

Oxford New York

Auckland Cape Town Dar es Salaam Hong Kong Karachi
Kuala Lumpur Madrid Melbourne Mexico City Nairobi
New Delhi Shanghai Taipei Toronto

With offices in

Argentina Austria Brazil Chile Czech Republic France Greece
Guatemala Hungary Italy Japan Poland Portugal Singapore
South Korea Switzerland Thailand Turkey Ukraine Vietnam

Oxford is a registered trade mark of Oxford University Press
in the UK and in certain other countries

Published in the United States
by Oxford University Press, Inc., New York

British Library Cataloguing in Publication Data
Data available

Library of Congress Cataloging in Publication Data
Data available

Typeset by Newgen Imaging Systems (P) Ltd., Chennai, India
Printed in Italy
on acid-free paper by Legoprint S.p.A

ISBN 0–19–857078–3 (Flexicover: alk.paper)
     978–0–19–857078–3 (Flexicover: alk.paper)

10 9 8 7 6 5 4 3 2 1

9/19/07

Foreword

The first legislation allowing nurses to prescribe was enacted in 1992. It empowered District Nurses and Health Visitors to prescribe from a very restricted formulary. Even so, implementation was cautious and the national roll out came only in 1998. Since then, developments have been much more rapid so that now suitably trained and experienced nurses can prescribe from the entire National Formulary. The whole nursing profession—clinicians, educators, managers and regulators—have worked together to ensure the success of this extension of practice. In some areas, they have set new standards for prescribing practice. The anxieties that were expressed at the outset have proved to be unfounded, confidence has been built up, and the experience with nurse prescribing has informed the subsequent implementation of prescribing powers for other health professions.

The authority to prescribe has enabled nurses to use their skills more effectively and to take responsibility for their own clinical decisions. It has allowed professional teams to develop in new ways. Most important, it has improved the quality of service to patients. There is already evidence not just of greater convenience but also of improved clinical outcomes. It is encouraging that in this area there is such a sound basis for contributions to the Government's efforts to extend the choice that is offered to patients. As the population ages and the prevalence of chronic diseases increases, nurse prescribers will be central to successful prevention and long term management.

The publication of the *Oxford Handbook of Nurse Prescribing* is another landmark in this field and I am sure it will be welcomed by the increasing numbers of nurse prescribers. I have been privileged to play a small part in this exciting development in health care in the United Kingdom. I am grateful to all my nursing colleagues whose hard work and determination have made it succeed beyond my dreams.

Dr. June Crown CBE,
Chairman, Review of the Prescribing,
Supply and Administration of Medicines.

Preface

This handbook gives authoritative, practical, and essential guidance on all aspects of the complex practice of prescribing. Following the style of the successful Oxford Handbooks with topic areas covering one or two pages and cross-referenced to other applicable information within the book, information is readily available to aid decision making.

Nurse Prescribing, now referred to as non-medical prescribing, had its inception in Julia Cumberledge's 1986 Government report on neighbourhood nursing which acknowledged that some nurses were prescribing without a legal or professional authorization[1]. An Advisory group's report on Nurse Prescribing (1989)[2] converted her earlier recommendations into today's prescribing mandate which was given the royal assent in 1992. Later that year the Medicinal Products: Prescription by Nurses Act and the required secondary legislation were passed enabling the selection of eight demonstration sites and in 1994 eligible nurses (public health nurses, health visitors, and home/district nurses) received English Nursing Board (ENB) training in safe prescribing from a limited formulary.

Following successful evaluation by the Universities of Liverpool and York, a further expansion in 1996 included 60 more practices in England and two more pilot sites in Scotland. Publication of the white paper *Delivering the Future*[3] led to seven more pilot sites and then a national roll-out to 23,000 eligible practitioners who undertook the Mode 1 course (blended learning). Students undertaking a specialist practitioner's degree completed the Mode 2 preparation (a taught module).

Gaining pace and following two favourable evaluative reports by June Crown in 1999[4,5] and *The NHS Plan*[6] prescribing rights were extended to other groups of nurses as independent prescribers. By May 2001, the Nurse Prescribers, formulary and ENB training (V200) were extended for nurses, midwives, and health visitors to include four new prescribing areas:

- Minor illness
- Minor injuries
- Health promotion
- Palliative care.

1 Department of Health and Social Security (1986). *Neighbourhood nursing—a focus for care*. HMSO, London.
2 Department of Health (1989). *Report of the Advisory Group on Nurse Prescribing*. Department of Health, London.
3 Department of Health (1996). *Delivering the Future*. Department of Health, London.
4 Department of Health (1998). Review of prescribing, supply and administration of medicines. A report on the supply and administration of medicines under group protocols. Department of Health, London.
5 Department of Health (1999). Review of prescribing, supply and administration of medicines. Final report. Department of Health, London.
6 Department of Health (2000). *The NHS plan: a plan for investment, a plan for reform*. Department of Health, London.

The Nurse Prescribers' Extended Formulary (NPEF) included all pharmacy and general sales list (GSL) medicines and initially a list of 140 prescription-only items used for treating specific conditions in the four areas listed.

Extended, Supplementary, and Independent Prescribing (V300) qualification registered with the Nurses and Midwives Council (NMC) enabled supplementary prescribers to prescribe any medicines or controlled drugs as part of a clinical management plan (CMP).

The new standards for prescribing were introduced in May 2006[7] and it is anticipated that there will be changes to the NMC register to introduce standards for specialist practice.

Amendments to legislation in May 2006 enabled independent nurse prescribers to prescribe from anywhere in the British National Formulary for any medical condition within their competence with the exception of unlicensed drugs. Nurse Independent Prescribing by V300 nurse prescribers now includes some controlled drugs[8].

With each extension of prescribing areas, the practitioners prescribing knowledge base needs to develop and this handbook provides advice on all aspects of prescribing decision making: for novice and student alike, as well as for all prescribing courses and following all the competency areas.

---

7 Department of Health (2006). Improving patients' access to medicines: A guide to implementing nurse and pharmacist independent prescribing within the NHS in England. Department of Health, London.
8 Nursing and Midwifery Council (2006). Standards of proficiency for nurse and midwife prescribers. NMC, London.

Acknowledgements

We would like to thank our reviewers: Caroline Abbot, Elaine Broad-bridge, and Elaine Scott-Bown. Thanks also to Steve Emmett.

Special thanks go to Graham Brack for being a gentlemanly, critical friend.

Thanks also to Caroline Hardy for her initial input to the book.

This book is dedicated to William Beckwith, and Simon, Matt, and Andy Franklin.

Contributors

Graham Brack, Pharamaceutical Adviser, Central Cornwall PCT
Caroline Hardy, Lecturer, Oxford Brookes University

Contents

Detailed contents

Symbols and abbreviations

~	Approx
±	Plus/minus
↑	Increased
↓	Decreased
↔	Normal
1°	Primary
2°	Secondary
°	Degrees
📖	Cross reference
🖥	Internet site
ABPI	Ankle Brachial Pressure Index
ACE	Angiotensin converting enzyme
ADE	Adverse drug effect
ADI	Adverse drug interaction
ADR	Adverse drug reaction
AIDS	Acquired immune deficiency syndrome
ASTRO-PU	Adjusted for age, sex, temporary resident originated prescribing unit
BAN	British approved name
BDA	British Diabetic Association (now Diabetes UK)
BHF	British Heart foundation
BHS	British Hypertensive Society
BMJ	*British Medical Journal*
BNF	*British National Formulary*
BTS	British Thoracic Society
CAT	Critical appraisal trials
CG	Clinical governance
CHD	Coronary heart disease
CNS	Central nervous system
CMP	Clinical management plan
CPF	Nurse Prescribers' Formulary for community practitioners

CNS	Central nervous system
COC	Combined hormonal contraceptive
COPD	Chronic obstructive airways disease
CP	Community practitioner (who hold a community specialist practice qualification and who can prove that they will use prescribing in their practice).
CPD	Continuing professional development
CRAG	Clinical resource audit group
CSBS	Clinical Standards Board for Scotland
CSM	Committee on Safety of Medicines
CVD	Cardiovascular disease
CVA	Cerebrovascular accident (stroke)
DL	Distance learning
DN	District nurse
DNA	Deoxyribonucleic acid
DoH	Department of Health
DVLA	Drivers and Vehicle Licensing Authority
EBP	Evidence based practice
EPACT	Electronic prescribing analysis and cost
FAQ	Frequently asked questions
FSH	Follicle stimulating hormone
GFR	Glomerula filtration rate
GI	Gastrointestinal
GMC	General Medical Council
GP	General practitioner
GSL	General sales list
GTN	Glyceryl trinitrate
hCG	Chorionic gonadotrophin
HDL	High density lipoprotein
HEI	Higher education institute
HIV	Human immunodeficiency virus
HOWIS	Health of Wales
HRT	Hormone replacement therapy
HV	Health visitor
IDDM	Insulin dependent diabetes mellitus
IM	Intra muscular
INR	International normalized ratio
IUD	Inter-uterine device
IV	Intravenous

LA	Local anaestheitc
LDL	Low density lipoprotein
LH	Luteinizing hormone
LSD	Lysergide
MCA	Medicines control agency
MHRA	Medicines and Healthcare Products Regulatory Agency
MI	Myocardial infaction
MAOI	Monoamine oxidase inhibitor
MDMA	3,4-Methylenedioxymetamphetamine (ecstacy)
MSU	Mid-stream urine
NeLH	National electronic Library for Health
NCASP	National Clinical Audit Support Programme
NHS	National Health Service
NICE	National Institute of Clinical Excellence
NMC	Nursing and Midwifery Council
NPC	National precribing centre
NPEF	Nurse prescribers extended formulary
NSAID	Non-steroidal anti-inflammatory drug
NSF	National service framework
OSCE	Objective structured clinical examinations
OTC	Over the counter
P	Pharmacy only medicine
PACT	Prescribing analysis and cost
PASA	Purchasing and Supplies Agency
PCO	Primary Care Organization (formerly PCT)
PGD	Patient group direction
PID	Pelvic inflammatory disease
PMT	Pre-menstrual tension
POM	Prescription-only medicine
POP	Progesterone-only pill
PPA	Prescription pricing authority
PSD	Patient specific direction
PU	Prescribing unit
PVD	Peripheral vascular disease
RCN	Royal College Of Nurses
RHA	Regional Health Authority
rINN	Recommended international non-proprietary name
RNA	Ribonucleic acid
RTI	Renal tract infection

RTP	Return to practice
SAFF	Service financial framework
SCPHN	Specialist community public health nurse
SIGN	Scottish intercollegiate guidelines network
SPA	Scottish prescribing analysis
SPQ	Specialist practitioner qualification
SSRI	Selective serotonin reuptake inhibitor
STAR-PU	Specific therapeutic group, age, sex related prescribing unit
TENS	Transcutaneous electrical nerve stimulator
TDM	Therapeutic drug monitoring
UKMIPG	United Kingdom Medicines Information Pharmacists Group
UTI	Urinary tract infection
Vd	Volume of distribution
WHO	World Health Organization
Ml	Millilitre
PLI	Professional liability insurance
RCT	Randomized controlled trials
EVP	Evidence-based practice
OTC	Over the counter
UKMi	United Kingdom Medicines information service
UTI	Urinary tract infection
VAT	Value added tax

Glossary

Acquired immunity
Not present at birth. Either active or passive.

Active acquired immunity
Naturally acquired immunity following exposure to an antigen within the environment or induced active immunity following deliberate exposure to an antigen i.e. vaccination or immunization.

Adverse drug reaction (ADR)
A reaction related to the use of a specific drug or drugs which causes harm and/or discomfort beyond its predictable therapeutic effects, and which predictably may cause harm to the patient in the future if given in the smaller or larger dose or in the same dosage and regimen. With any ADR, treatment may warrant prevention of future reactions or alteration of the drug and dosage regimen and possible withdrawal of the product.

Adverse drug interation (ADI)
Alteration of the drug's effects by the prior or concurrent administration of another drug (drug–drug interactions) or by food (drug–food interactions).

Audit
An audit is a systematic and official examination of a record, process, structure, environment, or account to evaluate performance.

Black triangle drugs
These are new drugs. The black triangle indicates that their safety profile is being closely monitored.

CAMs
Complementary and alternative medicines. The treatment of disease using methods other than recognized/conventional medicine.

Change agent
A person skilled in the theory and implementation of planned change, who possesses well-developed leadership and management skills.

Clinical audit
Clinical audit is conducted by doctors (medical audit) and other health care professionals (nurses, physiotherapists, occupational therapists, speech therapists, etc.) and is the systematic critical analysis of the quality of clinical care.

Clinical management plan
The legal framework for supplementary prescribing.

Clinical supervision
This is a term used to describe a formal process of professional support and learning which enables practitioners to develop knowledge and competence, assume responsibility for their own practice, and enhance consumer protection and safety of care in complex situations.

Competent standard of care
Bolam Principle (1957): the nurse is required to act within her or his competency at all times and to exercise 'the ordinary skill of an ordinary "man" exercising that particular art', i.e. perform reasonably as practitioners trained to the same standard within the same/similar professions, within a recognized standard of competency.

Concordance
An informed partnership agreement which is negotiated between the prescriber and the patient.

Consent
To be valid, consent must be informed consent. Treating a patient without consent may constitute an assault and subject the nurse to damages for trespass to the person

Constipation (difficulty in passing stools)
Stools of poor bulk, sometimes caused by a diet low in fibre, or hardness, due to increased time in the intestine, or poor hydration—may be difficult to pass.

Controlled drugs
These are preparations that are subject to the Misuse of Drugs Regulations 2001 and are specified in schedules 2 and 3.

Diabetes
Diabetes mellitus is a chronic and progressive disease which alters the body's management of carbohydrate and fat metabolism. It is divided into Type 1 diabetes (previously known as insulin-dependant diabetes mellitus—IDDM) in which there is an absence of insulin, and Type 2 diabetes which is caused by the body's inefficient use of endogenous insulin (insulin resistance) and/or insufficient production of insulin.

Dispensing medication
An individual who is dispensing medicine may be preparing, supplying, or administering the medication to the patient. Good practice indicates that the dispenser acts as a second checker for the prescriber. When dispensing medication always adhere to local policy.

Drug Tariff
The Drug Tariff is produced monthly as a joint compilation between the Department of Health and the Prescription Pricing Authority.

Formualtion
The formulation of a medicine refers to its chemical and physical composition.

Innate immunity
This is present at birth and genetically determined. No relationship to exposure or innate immunity.

Nurse Prescribers' Formulary for Community Practitioners
Previously known as the Nurse Prescribers' Formulary (NPF).

Nurses and Midwives Council (NMC)
The professional regulatory body for nurses, midwives, and health visitors.

Overflow incontinence
The bladder overfills and urine leaks into the ureter. Symptoms include voiding small amounts of urine, hesitancy, poor flow, or post-micturition dribble. This condition may follow hysterectomy or be caused by faecal impaction, unwanted effects of a drug regimen, or prostatic hyperplasia.

PACT data
PACT (prescribing analysis and cost) and SPA (Scottish prescribing analysis) are available as audit reports of practitioners prescribing on a quarterly (3-monthly) basis. These data provide comparisons between local and national prescribing patterns and can be broken down to indicate individual prescribing patterns.

Palliative care
Prescribing for people who require palliative care involves the active total care and suppression of symptoms for those whose disease is not responsive to curative treatments. In addition to control of pain and other symptoms, it involves an holistic approach, embracing social, psychological, and spiritual dimensions.

Passive acquired immunity
Natural passive immunity following the transfer of antibodies from another person i.e., a mother to her baby either in utero, via the placenta or in breast milk; or induced passive immunity when antibodies are administered in the form of antisera to prevent or fight infection.

Patient-group directions (PGDs)
Written instructions to a specified range of health-care professionals for the sale, supply, and administration of medicines directly to groups of patients with specific, defined clinical conditions, who may not be individually identified before presentation for treatment. PGDs provide the legal framework for medicines to be given to groups of patients without prescriptions having to be written.

Patient-specific directions
These are written instructions from a doctor or dentist which are set out in the patient's notes (in primary care) and on the drug chart (in secondary care) to specified health-care professionals, instructing them to supply or administer medicines or appliances to a named patient. This might be a simple instruction in the patient's notes.

Pharmaid
Even BNFs which are 6–12 months old are of use for those working in developing countries.

The Commonwealth Pharmaceutical Association has a scheme, Pharmaid, which despatches older BNFs, in the month of November, to areas where they may be of use.

Public health
Public health is defined by Acheson as 'the science and art of preventing disease, prolonging life and promoting health through the organized efforts of society'.

Randomized controlled trial (RCT)
Study design where treatment, interventions, or enrolment into different study groups are assigned by random allocation.

If the sample size is large enough this design avoids bias and confounding variables.

Red flag
A system of identification for any significantly dangerous symptoms.

Social determinants of health
A person's ability to attain a standard of health and well-being is influenced by their genetic make up and their lifestyle choices.

Specific immunity
Provided by the lymphocytes, both T and B cells act as a coordinated response to specific antigens. T cells are responsible for the mediation of cell immunity providing defence against abnormal cells and pathogens inside cells. B cells respond to antigens and pathogens in body fluids providing humeral or antibody-mediated immunity.

Stress incontinence
An involuntary urine leak when abdominal pressure increases during physical activity, e.g. exercise or coughing. It is usually caused by muscular damage to the bladder outlet because of weakness of the pelvic floor musculature. Often precipitated by childbirth, post-menopausal oestrogen deficiency or as a complication following prostatic surgery

Supplementary prescribing
Supplementary prescribing is a voluntary prescribing partnership between the independent prescriber (doctor or dentist) and a supplementary prescriber, to implement an agreed patient-specific clinical management plan (CMP) with the patient's agreement.

Therapeutic range/index
This is a range within which plasma concentrations will be related to therapeutic effect

Urge incontinence
This is caused by instability of the detrusor muscle, or hyperreflexia, which causes the bladder to contract at times other than intended urination. The bladder may not empty completely and a residual volume greater than 100 ml is common. The cause is unknown but it may be due to obstruction or neurological disease.

Urinary incontinence
An involuntary or inappropriate loss of urine which can be demonstrated objectively.

Vicarious liability
An employer is vicariously liable for their employee's negligent acts or omissions in the course of employment, whether authorized or not, unless the employer can show that the employee was undertaking a frolic of his own rather than the employer's business. The individual nurse still carries responsibility and, as such, is accountable for his or her actions.

Yellow card
Yellow card reporting is the reporting of adverse reactions for any drug given to patients in UK to the Medicines and Health Care Products Regulatory Agency (MHRA).

Part I

Introduction

What is a nurse prescriber?

Nurse prescribing history and policy in context

Health is a devolved sphere of government and therefore policy and implementation may vary between England, Scotland, Wales, and Northern Ireland. However, the following imperatives can be applied to all countries within the United Kingdom.

Context
- Renegotiation of divisions in health-care labour
- Changing professional boundaries[1,2]
- Supports the ethos of the new and modern NHS[3]
- Expansion of nursing roles
- Introduction of nurse-led clinics
- Supports the nurse practitioner role[4].

Impact on practice
- Multidisciplinary teamwork approach to care[5–7]
- Wide range of clinical and geographical settings
- Blurring of traditional roles and practices.

Outcome for patients
- Patient choice and convenience[2,8]
- Patient-centred care
- Structured around need
- Appropriate, timely, effective, and cost-effective intervention
- Give consideration to best practice based on evidence[9]
- Nurses managing chronic disease.

Caution
Practice with caution and awareness of the necessity to prescribe:
- within the limitations of competencies
- to the required legal framework.[10]

📖 Seven principles of safe prescribing.

1 Department of Health (1999). *Making a difference: strengthening the nursing, midwifery and health visiting contribution to health and healthcare.* DoH, London.

2 Department of Health (2002). *Liberating the talents: helping Primary Care Trusts and nurses to deliver the NHS Plan.* DoH, London.

3 Department of Health (2000). *The NHS Plan: a plan for investment, a plan for reform.* DoH, London.

4 Baird, A. (2001). Diagnosis and prescribing: the impact of nurse prescribing on professional roles. *Primary Health Care*, **11**, 24–6.

5 Her Majesty's Stationary Office (1994). *Medicinal Products Prescription by Nurses etc Act* (Commencement No. 1). HMSO, London.

6 Her Majesty's Stationary Office (2001). *Health and Social Care Act.* HMSO, London.

7 Her Majesty's Stationary Office (2003). *The Prescription Only Medicines (Human Use) Amendment Order.* HMSO, London.

8 Department of Health (2004). *Choosing Health: making healthier choices easier.* DoH, London.

9 Latter, S. and Courtney, M. (2004). Effectiveness of nurse prescribing: a review of the literature. *Journal of Clinical Nursing*, **13**(1), 26–32.

10 Humphries, J.L. and Green, J. (2002). *Nurse prescribing*, 2nd edn. Palgrave, Basingstoke.

Further reading

Department of Health (2005). *Non-medical prescribing: supplementary prescribng of controlled drugs (nurses and pharmacists)*. DoH, London.

Student nurse prescribers and methods of training

Prescribing training

This training is accessed through the clinical leads of Primary Care Organizations (PCOs) and NHS trusts. The courses are funded by the Strategic Health Authority (SHA) work force development directorates. Each SHA has a non-medical prescribing lead.

Mode 1

This training, the original nurse prescribing, is available for district nurses (DNs) and health visitors (HVs) who are in post.

- It consists either of a half day introductory session followed by a 6 week self-directed distance learning (DL) pack with 3 taught consolidation days or:
- Attendance at a Higher Education Institute (HEI) for the Nurse Prescribing Module which is part of the Specialist Practitioner degree award.
- Either type of mode 1 is assessed by a two-part examination: part 1, a short answer paper, is followed by a second paper which looks at prescribing issues in greater depth.
- Generally eight level 3 (undergraduate level) CAT points are awarded on successful completion of mode 1, although there are some variations in assessment techniques from one HEI to another.

Mode 2

This is the mode of training undertaken by students studying for a community specialist practice qualification (SPQ) as part of a specialist practitioner degree award.

- It is a taught module assessed at level 3 by a written case study (vignette) and by completed competencies in practice.
- Fifteen level 3 CAT points are generally awarded on successful completion of this module.

Nurse Independent and Supplementary Prescribing formally Nurse Independent Prescribing (V300)

This mode of study is open to all registered nurses who are identified by their managers as having the type of practice where their ability to prescribe would enhance patient care.

Following this additional training, nurses who are working within their competencies may prescribe from anywhere within the BNF, including a list of controlled drugs and with the exception of unlicensed medicines.

The students also need to demonstrate an ability to study at level 3:

- This is a taught course with 26 full days spent at university and 12 days spent in practice with a designated medical practitioner (a doctor).
- It is usually assessed at level 3 by an examination comprising one short and one long answer paper, a portfolio, the completion of competencies in practice, and an objective structured clinical examination (OSCE). There are some variations in assessment techniques from one HEI to another.
- Generally twenty level 3 CAT points are awarded on successful completion although there are some variations in assessment techniques from one HEI to another.
- Some universities offer this course as *blended learning* with the addition of a distance learning component.

Supplementary Prescribing (V300)

Supplementary prescribing

Definition of supplementary prescribing (formally known as dependent prescribing):

> A voluntary partnership between an independent prescriber, (a doctor or dentist) and a supplementary prescriber to implement an agreed patient specific Clinical Management Plan (CMP) with the patient's agreement.[1]

Supplementary nurse prescribers are:
- Selected locally and must have opportunities to prescribe in the post occupied on completion of prescribing training.
- Able to demonstrate an ability to study at level 3.
- Able to demonstrate 3 years post registration clinical experience.
- Able to prescribe any medicines and controlled drugs that are listed in an agreed Clinical Management Plan (CMP).
- Able to prescribe controlled drugs because of amendments to the Misuse of Drugs regulations 2001 and to the GMS/PMS regulations which came into effect on 14 April 2005.
- Examples of CMPs may be obtained from www.dh.gov.uk/ PolicyAndGuidance/MedicinesPharmacyAndIndustry/ Prescriptions/SupplementaryPrescribing/fs/en

For Supplementary Prescribing Independent Prescribers

Must be doctors or dentists.
- Will discuss with supplementary prescribers which patients may benefit from supplementary prescribing and which medicines may be included in a CMP.
- Should be responsible for the patient's care.
- Are responsible for making the diagnosis and setting the parameters for the CMP.
- The supplementary prescriber has discretion regarding the frequency, dose, and product in addition to other variables outlined within the CMP.
- It is essential that there is clarity regarding the prescribing regimen being used i.e. community practitioner nurse prescribers or a nurse independent prescriber or a supplementary prescriber.

Supplementary prescribing training

To qualify as a supplementary nurse prescriber a nurse also has to train as an independent nurse prescriber.

Nurse independent prescribing

The *Nurse Prescribers Extended Formulary* (NPEF) ceased to exist in May 2006 when amendments to legislation enabled nurse independent prescibers to prescribe any licensed medicine with the inclusion of some controlled drugs which are listed in the BNF and Drug Tariff and by the Department of Health[1]. Nurse Independent Prescribers must not prescribe unless they have assessed their patient and are clinically competent[2].

This extension means that specialist nurses running diabetes and coronary heart disease clinics will be able to prescribe independently for their patients. Pharmacists will be able to prescribe independently for the local community; for example, controlling high blood pressure, smoking cessation, diabetes, etc. This will take pressure off GPs, allowing them to focus on more complex cases and improving the availability of care for patients.[2]

Supplementary prescribing

Supplementary prescribing in partnership with a doctor or dentist independent prescriber will continue for the management of complex conditions and for shared care.

Patient group directions (PGDs)

There are no special training requirements for nurses and pharmacists who supply and administer medicines through the use of a PGD. However, the National Prescribing Centre (NPC) suggest that those using PGDs should receive at least one day's training in their use provided at local level and yearly updates.

The NPC have developed a competency framework to guide development and training at a local level and this may be accessed on: ⊟ http://www.npc.co.uk/non_medical.htm

1 DoH (2006). *Improving Patients' Access to Medicines: A guide to Implementing Nurse and Pharmacist Independent Prescribing Within the NHS in England.* DoH, London
2 Nursing and Midwifery Council (2006). *Standard of Proficiency for nurse and midwife prescribers.* NMC. London.

Timeline for nurse prescribing

1968	Medicines Act
1986	Neighbourhood Nursing: a Focus for Care
1989	First Crown Report
1992	Medicinal Products: Prescription by Nurses Act
1994	Medicinal Products Prescription by Nurses etc. Act (Commencement No. 1)
1999	Second Crown Report (Crown Review)
2000	Consultation on proposals to extend nurse prescribing
2000	Freedom of Information Act
2001	Health and Social Care Act
2003	Amendments to the Prescription Only Medicines Order and NHS regulations
2006	Nurse Independent prescribing
2006	Introduction of Nursing and Midwifery Council standards for prescribing

1968 Medicines Act

Covered the establishment of the medical agency; the manner and type of licence needed for research on medicinal products, the manufacture, import, and storage of medicines, and, of particular relevance to nursing and midwifery, the manner in which medicines can be supplied and administered by health professionals such as doctors, pharmacists, nurses, and midwives.

1986 Neighbourhood Nursing: a Focus for Care

Report of the Community Nursing Review, the Cumberledge Report. Recommended limited prescribing rights for community nurses with district nurse or health visitor qualifications.

1989 First Crown Report

Report on the Advisory Group on Nurse Prescribing. Recommended nurse prescribers and other professionals as prescribers for the future enhancement of patient care.

1992 Medicinal Products: Prescription by Nurses Act

Primary legislation: royal assent to limited prescribing rights for health visitors, district nurses, and practice nurses with a health visiting or district nursing qualification.

1994 Medicinal Products Prescription by Nurses etc. Act (Commencement No. 1)

Secondary legislation enabling health visitors, district nurses, and practice nurses with a health visiting or district nursing qualification to prescribe.

1999 Second Crown Report (Crown Review)
Review of prescribing, supply, and administration of medicines. Recommended the supply and administration of medicines under group protocols for nurses and other professionals.

2000 Consultation on proposals to extend nurse prescribing
This included extending the scope of nurse prescribing, which does not require primary legislation, and also extending prescribing rights to other health professionals.

2000 Freedom of Information Act
This Act gives the public the right to view information held in the public domain by public authorities such as the NHS. This includes prescribing policies and protocols. The handling and disclosure of personal regulation is exempted and is regulated by the Data Protection Act 1998.

2001 Health and Social Care Act
Provided necessary legislation for the implementation of independent extended nurse prescribing. Nurses were given the rights to prescribe independently from an extended nurse prescribing formulary.

2003 Amendments to the Prescription Only Medicines Order and NHS regulations
Allowed supplementary prescribing by suitably trained nurses and pharmacists.

Spring 2005 amendments to the Prescription Only Medicines Order and NHS regulations
Allowed Supplementary prescribing of controlled drugs by nurses and pharmacists in primary and secondary care.

2006 Nurse Independent Prescribing
From May 2006, the Nurse Prescribers' Extended Formulary was discontinued and qualified nurse independent prescribers (formally known as extended formulary nurse prescribers) were able to prescribe any licensed medicine for any medical conditions within their competence, including some controlled drugs.

From Spring 2006 the name of the Nurse Prescribers' Formulary (for V100 prescribers) was changed to the Nurse Practitioners' Formulary for Community Practitioners. Nurses who undertake mode 2 training as part of a community specialist practice qualification (SPQ) are licensed with the Nursing and Midwifery Council to prescribe from this formulary.

Spring 2006: introduction of the Nursing and Midwifery Council's Standards of Proficiency for Nurse and Midwife prescribers (NMC, 2006)

The legal differences between prescribing, administering, and dispensing

Administration of drugs

Administration of drugs can occur as a result of a patient-group direction (PGD) or a written patient-specific direction (PSD) of which a prescription is one example.

PGDs

Recommended by the Second Crown Report,[1] patient-group direction is legal terminology for what used to be known as group protocols.

PGDs provide written instructions to a specified range of health-care professionals for the sale, supply, and administration of medicines directly to groups of patients with specific, defined clinical conditions, who may not be individually identified before presentation for treatment.[2] PGDs provide the legal framework for medicines to be given to groups of patients without prescriptions having to be written.

Medication can be administered by specified health professionals under a PGD without them necessarily having to consult with a prescriber, and without the patient necessarily seeing a prescriber. Responsibility for assessment to ascertain whether the patient fits the criteria within the PGD lies with the health professional.

PGDs are not designed to manage long-term/chronic conditions. Management of such conditions is best achieved by a health-care professional prescribing for the individual patient.

Legal framework for PGDs
• The Prescription Only Medicines (Human Use) Amendment Order 2000[3].
• The Medicine (Pharmacy and General Sale – Exemption) Amendment Order 2000[4].
• The Medicines (Sale and Supply) (Miscellaneous Provisions) Amendment (No 2) Regulations 2000[5].

A senior doctor or dentist and pharmacist must provide signed authorization for a PGD; they must also have been instrumental in developing the PGD. The PGD must be ratified by the Trust or organization through governance.

1 Department of Health (1999) *Review of prescribing, supply and administration of medicines: Final report.* DoH, London.
2 Department of Health (2004) *Policy and Guidance: Patient Group Directions (PGD)?* 🖫 http://www.dh.gov.uk/PolicyAndGuidance/EmergencyPlanning/EmergencyPreparednessArticle/fs/en?CONTENT_ID=4069610&chk=in7ZEF
3 Her Majesty's Stationary Office (2000) *The Prescription Only Medicines (Human Use) Amendment Order 2000.* HMSO, London.
4 Her Majesty's Stationary Office (2000) *The Medicine (Pharmacy and General Sale—Exemption) Amendment Order 2000.* HMSO, London.
5 Her Majesty's Stationary Office (2000) *The Medicines (Sale and Supply) (Miscellaneous Provisions) Amendment (No 2) Regulations 2000.* HMSO, London.

Qualified health professionals who, provided they are named individuals, can sell, supply, or administer medicines under a PGD include:
• nurses
• midwives
• health visitors
• optometrists
• pharmacists
• chiropodists
• radiographers
• orthoptists
• physiotherapists
• ambulance paramedics
• dietitians
• occupational therapists
• speech and language therapists
• prosthetists
• orthotists.

Appropriate settings for use of PGDs

Areas where a patient has not been already identified, for example:
• minor injury clinics
• minor illness clinics
• first contact services
• out of hours services
• emergency situations
• family planning clinics
• immunization clinics.

Patient-specific directions

These are written instructions from a doctor or dentist which are set out in the patient's notes (in primary care) and on the drug chart (in secondary care) to specified health-care professionals, instructing them to supply or administer medicines or appliances to a named patient. This might be a simple instruction in the patient's notes.

Dispensing medication

An individual who is dispensing medicine may be preparing, supplying, or administering the medication to the patient. Good practice indicates that the dispenser acts as a second checker for the prescriber. When dispensing medication always adhere to local policy.

Nursing and Midwifery Council (NMC) Code of Professional Conduct: standards of conduct, performance, and ethics

The NMC is the professional regulatory body for nurses, midwives, and health visitors.

Background

- The Code of Professional Conduct was published by the Nursing and Midwifery Council (NMC) in April 2002 and came into effect on 1 June 2002.
- It replaced the United Kingdom Central Council for Nursing, Midwifery, and Health Visiting Code of Conduct.
- In August 2004 an addendum was published and the name was changed to NMC Code of Professional Conduct: standards of conduct, performance, and ethics.
- All references to 'nurses, midwives, and health visitors' were replaced by 'nurses, midwives, and public health nurses'.
- A new section on indemnity insurance was added and the updated version of the code was published in November 2004.[1]

Summary

As a registered nurse, midwife, or specialist community public health nurse, you must:
- respect the patient or client as an individual
- obtain consent before you give any treatment or care
- cooperate with others in the team
- protect confidential information
- maintain your professional knowledge and competence
- be trustworthy
- act to identify and minimize the risk to patients and clients.

Prescribing and the implications of delegation[1]

The NMC has set out guidelines for the administration of medicines.[2] The prescriber is responsible for (accountable for):
- record keeping, even if the administration is delegated
- ensuring that the prescribed/recommended item is applied or administered as directed, either by the patients, their carers, the nurse his/herself, or any other person to whom the task is delegated.

Delegation must not compromise existing care and must serve the needs and interests of the patients or clients (NMC 2004, Section 4.6).[1]

---

1 Nursing and Midwifery Council (2004). *Code of professional conduct: standards for conduct, performance and ethics.* ⬛ Available on the NMC website at www.nmc-uk.org, and printed copies can be obtained from: publications@nmc-uk.org

2 Nursing and Midwifery Council (2004). *Guidelines for the administration of medicines.* NMC, London. ⬛ Available at www.nmc-uk.org/nmc/main/publications/Guidelinesformedicines.pdf

Prescribing and co-operation with others in the team

NMC code Section 4 states you must co-operate with others in the team.[1] The team comprises:
- patient or client and their family
- informal carers
- health and social care professionals in the NHS
- those in the independent and voluntary sectors.

Cooperation includes:
- respecting the expertise and skills of colleagues
- treating them fairly and without discrimination
- communicating effectively; use of health-care records
- sharing knowledge, skills, and expertise
- cooperating with internal and external investigations (NMC 2004, Section 4.7).[1]

Section 2

Principles

Principles of supplementary prescribing

What is supplementary prescribing?

Supplementary prescribing is a voluntary prescribing partnership between the independent prescriber (doctor or dentist) and a supplementary prescriber, to implement an agreed patient-specific clinical management plan (CMP) with the patient's agreement.[1]

Rationale for supplementary prescribing

- Maximum benefit to patients.
- Patient choice of prescriber.
- Flexible use of workforce.
- For patients with multiple health needs or multiple professional carers.
- Works well for the management of chronic conditions.
- May not be suitable for all cases.
- The independent prescriber can decide as to suitability of implementation of a CMP.

Legislation

- The 1998 Crown 2 Review of Prescribing — suggested widening prescribing rights to enable nurses and some allied health professionals to prescribe from patient group directions and as dependent prescribers.
- Dependent prescribing changed to supplementary prescribing.
- Section 63 of the Health and Social Care Act 2001 — designated new categories of prescriber with set conditions.
- Amendments to prescription only medicines order (2003).
- Changes to NHS regulations.
- Enforced (April 2003).
- 📖 Timeline for nurse prescribing.

Who can qualify as a supplementary prescriber?

Registered:

- nurses
- pharmacists
- optometrists
- podiatrists
- physiotherapists
- radiographers.

Key principles

- Patient safety is paramount.
- Patient appropriate and patient specific.
- Only prescribe within competency area.
- Independent prescriber makes the diagnosis.
- Independent prescriber must be a doctor (or dentist).
- Voluntary partnership.

---

1 Department of Health (2005) Supplementary Prescribing by Nurses, Pharmacists, Chiropodists/Podiatrists, Physiotherapists and Radiographers within the NHS in England: A Guide for Implementation – updated May 2005. DoH, London.

- Patient agreement paramount.
- CMPs could refer to appropriate reputable guidelines or agreed protocols for treatment of a specific condition.
- Guidelines/protocols should be easily available for the supplementary prescriber.
- Supplementary prescribing can include a team approach to prescribing with more than one independent and supplementary prescriber who is signed up to the plan.
- Communication between all prescribers of primacy.
- Shared access to the patient record.
- Supports multidisciplinary care.
- CMP needs to be simple otherwise it won't happen.

Practice specific to supplementary prescribing

General principles of supplementary prescribing, as listed below, apply to prescribing in both acute and primary care.

CMPs need to be set up for the patient with the patient's knowledge in advance of any nurse prescribing.

- Ensure that a voluntary prescribing agreement has been negotiated between the independent prescriber(s), the patient, and the supplementary prescriber(s).
- Prescribe within your competency area.
- Always inform the patient/carer of prescribing actions.
- Gain consent from the patient/carer.
- Ensure that all parties have access to the CMP.
- Communicate all prescribing decisions with other prescribers who are involved in the patient's care.
- Where possible, use shared electronic records.
- Where there is co-terminus access to records, use the template as illustrated.
- Where there is no access to co-terminus records, use the template as illustrated.
- Templates can be established for the treatment of specific conditions (however these must be adapted to meet the needs of the individual patient).

Template CMP 1 (blank): for teams that have full co-terminus access to patient records

Name of patient:		Patient medication sensitivities/allergies:		
Patient identification e.g. ID number, date of birth:				
Independent prescriber(s):		Supplementary prescriber(s)		
Condition(s) to be treated		Aim of treatment		
Medicines that may be prescribed by SP:				
Preparation	Indication	Dose schedule	Specific indications for referral back to the IP	
Guidelines or protocols supporting Clinical Management Plan:				
Frequency of review and monitoring by:				
Supplementary prescriber:				
Supplementary prescriber and independent prescriber:				
Process for reporting ADRs:				
Shared record to be used by IP and SP:				
Agreed by independent pre-scriber(s)	Date	Agreed by sup-plementary pre-scriber(s)	Date	Date agreed with patient/carer

Reproduced with permission from the Department of Health.

Template CMP 2 (blank): for teams where the SP does not have co-terminus access to the medical record

Name of patient:		Patient medication sensitivities/allergies:		
Patient identification e.g. ID number, date of birth:				
Current medication:		Medical history:		
Independent prescriber(s):		Supplementary prescriber(s):		
Contact details: [tel/email/address]		Contact details: [tel/email/address]		
Condition(s) to be treated:		Aim of treatment:		
Medicines that may be prescribed by SP:				
Preparation	Indication	Dose schedule	Specific indications for referral back to the IP	
Guidelines or protocols supporting Clinical Management Plan:				
Frequency of review and monitoring by:				
Supplementary prescriber :				
Supplementary prescriber and independent prescriber:				
Process for reporting ADRs:				
Shared record to be used by IP and SP:				
Agreed by independent prescriber(s)	Date	Agreed by supplementary prescriber(s)	Date	Date agreed with patient/carer

Reproduced with permission from the Department of Health.

Supplementary prescribing within the acute sector

In the acute sector you may use an adapted version of the hospital prescribing sheet as long as it is line with local policy or an FP10.
• Ensure that the hospital pharmacy has a record of your signature.

Some examples of clinical conditions where supplementary prescribing can be used in the acute setting
• Stroke management
• Erythropoiesis
• Pain management
• Palliative care
• Cardiology
• Oncology
• Diabetes
• Hypertension
• Chronic obstructive pulmonary disease
• Asthma
• Paediatrics
• Cystic fibrosis.

📖 Writing a clinical management plan.

Own examples of prescribing within the acute sector

Supplementary prescribing in the primary care setting

The same general principles apply for supplementary prescribing in the primary care sector as in the acute sector.

Practice specific to prescribing in primary care
- Provide community pharmacies with a copy of your signature.
- Prescribe from FP10 Independent Supplementary prescriber prescription.
- Ensure that your contact number and budget code are indicated on the prescription.

Examples of clinical conditions for which supplementary prescribing can be used in the primary care setting
- Smoking cessation
- Chronic obstructive pulmonary disease
- Asthma
- Chronic eczema/skin complaints
- Hypertension
- Diabetes.

Further reading

📖 Department of Health (2006) http://www.dh.gov.uk/PolicyAndGuidance/MedicinesPharmacy
AndIndustry/Prescriptions/NonmedicalPrescribing/Supplementary
Prescribing/SupplementaryPrescribingArticle/fs/en?CONTENT_ID=4123030&chk=t3E8Fk

Own examples of prescribing within the primary care setting

Clinical management plans

What is a clinical management plan?

A clinical management plan (CMP) is an agreed, defined plan of treatment for a named patient which sets the legal boundaries of the medication and the parameters of prescribing responsibility for the supplementary prescriber. The plan must be agreed as a result of a voluntary partnership between the independent doctor or dentist prescriber and the supplementary prescriber, and with the knowledge of the patient and/or carer (📖 Supplementary prescribing).

Only qualified supplementary prescribers who hold a recordable qualification, as recognized by their regulatory body (in the case of nurses, the NMC) can prescribe as supplementary prescribers. Supplementary prescribers must only prescribe within their clinical field of competence. A CMP:
- is the legal framework for supplementary prescribing
- is a plan of care that relates specifically to a named patient and the specific condition(s) to be managed
- must be in place before prescribing.
📖 Supplementary prescribing.
📖 Practical examples of CMPs.

What must be included on a CMP?
- The name of the patient to whom the plan relates.
- The illness or conditions which may be treated by the supplementary prescriber.
- The date on which the plan is to start.
- The date when the plan is to be reviewed by the independent prescriber.
- The date of review by the supplementary prescriber.
- The class or description of medicines or appliances which may be prescribed or administered under the plan.
- Restrictions or limitations of strength or dose of medicines which may be prescribed or administered under the plan.
- The period of administration or use of medicines or appliances which may be prescribed or administered under the plan.
- Relevant warnings about known sensitivities of the patient to medicines or appliances.
- Known difficulties the patient has with particular medicines or appliances.
- The arrangements for notification of:
  - suspected or known reactions to any medicine which may be prescribed or administered according to the plan
  - suspected or known adverse reactions to any other medicine taken at the same time as any medicine prescribed or administered under the plan
  - incidents occurring with the appliance which might lead, might have led to or has led to the death or serious deterioration of the state of health of the patient
  - circumstances in which the supplementary prescriber should refer to, or seek the advice of the independent prescriber or prescribers who are party to the plan.
- Date for review—at least annual, and more often where needed[1].

1 Department of Health (2003) *Guidelines: Supplementary Prescribing: frequently asked quesions.* 🖳 Available from www.doh.gov.uk/supplementaryprescribing

How can supplementary prescribing be effectively implemented into practice?
- CMPs have to be relatively simple and quick to complete.
- A plan should not duplicate information already in the shared record.

Communication
- Is vital between independent prescriber(s) and supplementary prescriber(s).
- Remote partnerships work best when there are shared electronic records
- The CMP should include national and local guidelines which must clearly identify the range of the relevant medicinal products to be used in the treatment of the patient
- The CMP should draw attention to the relevant part of the guideline
- Guidelines referred to need to be easily accessible

Further reading
Department of Health (2005) *Supplementary Prescribing by Nurses, Pharmacists, Chiropodists/ Podiatrists, Physiotherapists and Radiographers within the NHS in England, May 2005.* Available from www.doh.gov.uk/supplementaryprescribing

Developing, writing, and implementing a CMP

Developing a CMP

The agreed written plan must be in place before prescribing begins. There are two types of template on which CMPs can be written:

- The first is designed for situations where all of the prescribers who are involved in the management of the case have full co-terminus access to patient records (Template CMP 1).
- The second is designed for teams and can be used where the supplementary prescriber does not have co-terminus access to the medical record (Template CMP 2).

Writing a CMP

- There are no legal restrictions on the clinical conditions which can be treated or on what can be prescribed as a result of a CMP.
- All conditions which have previously (before the implementation of supplementary prescribing) been prescribed for by an independent doctor or dentist prescriber can be treated and prescribed for by a supplementary prescriber under the umbrella of an agreed CMP.
- Wherever possible, the CMP must cite national and locally agreed guidelines.
- The prescriber must (wherever possible) adhere to agreed local and national guidelines.

Essential information

When writing a CMP one should always include:

- the name of the patient
- the condition(s) to be treated
- class and/or description of medication(s)
- dose ranges and strengths
- range restrictions
- timescale over which the medication is to be given
- refer to local and national guidelines
- allergies and sensitivities to medication(s) or other substances
- how to report allergies and sensitivities
- when and why to refer back to the independent prescriber(s)
- keep the plan appropriately simple
- write the plan in a language that everyone can understand.

What can be prescribed?

Supplementary prescribers, when working to an agreed clinical management plan, can prescribe:

- all general sales list (GSL) medicines, pharmacy (P) medicines, appliances and devices, foods, and other borderline substances approved by the Advisory Committee on Borderline Substances
- all prescription-only medicines for use outside of their licensed indications (i.e. 'off label' prescribing), 'black triangle' drugs, and drugs marked 'less suitable for prescribing' in the BNF

- unlicensed drugs
- supplementary prescribers are advised to prescribe generically except where not clinically indicated (e.g in the case of a drug with a specific bioavailability) or when the product does not have an approved generic name.

When is supplementary prescribing best used?

- Supplementary prescribing is the most useful method for prescribing when the patient's condition requires them to be treated with unlicensed medication.
- Medication which is outside of its product licence, e.g smoking cessation products for teenagers.
- For controlled drugs which are not permitted by nurse independent prescribing.
- For complex conditions and shared care.

Practical examples of CMPs

Nurses can prescribe controlled drugs, unlicensed drugs, and drugs which are used for indications which are outside of their product licence as supplementary prescribers.

Supplementary prescribing is useful in specific cases for the management of chronic conditions, palliative care, and shared nurse/doctor care.

The following examples are taken from the inpatient care of a person with diabetes, palliative care of a person in the terminal stages of life, and public health nursing.

• **Template CMP 1:** CMP for inpatient care of a person with diabetes.
• **Template CMP 2:** CMP for care of a patient in the end stage of life (reproduced with acknowledgement to Michael Thomas, clinical nurse specialist in palliative care, Cornwall).
• **Template CMP 3:** CMP for care of a client who wishes to stop smoking.

Template CMP 1: for teams that have full co-terminus access to patient records

Name of patient: Mary Smith	Patient medication sensitivities/allergies: None known

Patient identification e.g. ID number, date of birth: 20.10.35

Independent prescriber(s): Dr F Bloggs (Consultant Diabetologist)	Supplementary prescriber(s) John Jones Inpatient Diabetic Nurse Specialist
Condition(s) to be treated	**Aim of treatment**
Type 2 Diabetes (steroid induced)	Normoglycaemia To optimize glycaemic control thereby minimizing risk of long-term complications To support patient in self management of diabetes

Medicines that may be prescribed by SP:

Preparation	Indication	Dose schedule	Specific indications for referral back to the iP
Pre-mixed insulin 30/70 and appropriate delivery system	To achieve normal glycaemia	As indicated by clinical need (see appropriate section BNF)	Unsatisfactory blood glucose levels Significant hypoglycaemia

Guidelines or protocols supporting clinical management plan: Consult with local guidelines

NIHCE Guidelines for the Management of type 2 Diabetes: Management of Blood Glucose 2002

National Service Framework for Diabetes Mellitus (DOH, 2001)

Frequency of review and monitoring by:

Supplementary prescriber : Four hourly blood sugars as inpatient. On discharge initially daily by telephone contact until stable. Continue monitoring while steroid doses are reduced.

Supplementary prescriber and independent prescriber: Monitored by GP diabetic clinic unless further outpatient clinic required.

Process for reporting ADRs: Yellow card scheme to committee of safety of medicines and in patients shared electronic records. Report to Independent prescriber and to patient's GP

Shared record to be used by IP and SP:
Patient's medical notes.

Agreed by independent prescriber(s)	Date	Agreed by supplementary prescriber(s)	Date	Date agreed with patient/carer
Dr F Bloggs	20.03.06	John Jones	20.03.06	Mary Smith 20.03.06

Template CMP 2: for teams that have full co-terminus access to patient records

Name of Patient:	Patientmedication sensitivities/allergies:
James Bloggs	Nil known

Patient identification e.g. ID number, date of birth: 12. 09. 30

Independent Prescriber(s)	Supplementary Prescriber(s)
Dr K. Now	V. Kind

Condition(s) to be treated	Aim of treatment
Restlessness and agitation caused by breathlessness in the terminal stage of life	To reduce anxiety, sedate and induce amnesia

Medicines that may be prescribed by SP:

Preparation	Indication	Dose schedule	Specific indications for referral back to the IP
Midazolam	Restlessness and agitation as a result of terminal illness	15mg–30mg over 24 hrs (10mg in 2ml strength). Diluted with water for injections to 56mm via a continuous subcutaneous infusion via a Graseby MS26 pump	Paradoxical behaviour reactions Need for higher dose range to control symptoms

Guidelines or protocols supporting Clinical Management Plan:

www.palliativedrugs.com

Ellershaw, J (2003) Care of the dying

Stone, P et al. (1997) A comparison of the use of sedatives in a hospital support team and in a hospice

Bottomley, D. Hanks, G (1990). Subcutaneous Midazolam infusion for palliative care

Frequency of review and monitoring by:

Supplementary prescriber :Four hourly blood sugars as inpatient. On discharge initially daily by telephone contact until stable. Continue monitoring while steroid doses are reduced.

Supplementary prescriber and independent prescriber: Monitored by GP diabetic clinic unless further outpatient clinic required.

Process for reporting ADRs:

To Independent prescriber (Palliative Care Consultant)/ Patient's Consultant

Pharmacy Department/ Department/ Yellow card data system within the British National Formulary

Shared record to be used by IP and SP:

Patient's medical notes/Palliative care data system

Agreed by independent prescriber(s)	Date	Agreed by supplementary prescriber(s)	Date	Date agreed with patient/carer
Dr K Now	20.03.06	V Kind	20.03.06	20.03.06

Template CMP 3: for teams where the SP does not have co-terminus access to the medical record

Name of Patient: Lil Ashby	Patient medication sensitivities/allergies: None known or reported

Patient identification e.g. ID number, date of birth: 20.10.61	

Current medication: None	Medical history: Has a history of repeated chest infections. Patient has had two chest infections in the last six months. Patient smokes between 20 and 30 cigarettes a day.

Independent Prescriber(s): Dr Fred Bloggs Contact details: [tel/email/address] 98757428345	Supplementary prescriber(s): Penny Franklin Contact details: [tel/email/address] 01395 276483 pfranklin@eastenderspct.nhs.uk

Condition(s) to be treated: Nicotine dependency	Aim of treatment: To provide pharmaceutical support as part of a smoking cessation programme with view to supporting smoking cessation

Medicines that may be prescribed by SP:

Preparation	Indication	Dose schedule	Specific indications for referral back to the IP
As per East Lunghampton PCT fomulary Bupropion	Therapeutic support for smoking cessation in combination with motivational support	As per manufacturers summary of product characteristics (SPC), BNF page 248 and East Lunghampton PCT formulary pg 118	Increased adverse, common, uncommon and rare effects as indicated in summary of product characteristics: hypersensitivity reactions such as urticaria, sudden onset moderate to severe depression, sudden onset moderate to severe anxiety, chest pain, asthenia,tachycardia, increased blood pressure, confusion, anorexia, tinnitus, visual disturbance, vasodilation, syncope, seizures, moderate to severe irritability and hostility

Guidelines or protocols supporting Clinical Management Plan:
Guidance on the use of nicotine replacement therapy (NRT) and Buprorion for smoking cessation (National Institute for Clinical Excellence March 2002
Prodigy guidance and patient information leaflet – smoking cessation
(http://www.prodigy.nhs.uk/guidance.asp?gt= Smoking cessation

Frequency of review and monitoring by:
Supplementary prescriber : Weekly for first four weeks as indicated by response to treatment, and then 4, 6, 8 and 12 weekly
Supplementary prescriber and independent prescriber: Annually

Process for reporting ADRs:
Supplementary prescriber to report to Independent prescriber and to record in patient's records.
Notify by CSM yellow card system if indicated.

Shared record to be used by IP and SP:
Patient's EMIS electronic records.

Agreed by independent prescriber(s)	Date	Agreed by supplementary prescriber(s)	Date	Date agreed with patient/carer
Dr F Bloggs	20.02.05	Penny Franklin	20.02.05	21.02.05

Basic principles of pharmacology

Pharmacodynamics

Definition

Consideration of the effect a drug has on the body. Body functions are mediated by control systems which depend on:

- receptors on the cell surface
- carrier molecules
- enzymes
- specific macromolecules e.g. DNA.

Once drugs reach the area of their action they either work in a specific or non-specific manner.

Specific drug action

Interaction with receptors

Definition—a receptor

A receptor, usually a protein molecule, is found on the surface of a cell or is located inside a cell in the cytoplasm.

- Drugs interact with receptors forming a drug–receptor complex.
- A drug requires a complementary structure in order for it to interact with a receptor, i.e. lock and key model.
- Few drugs need a specific receptor and many will combine with more than one type of receptor.
- Drugs often display an affinity for one particular receptor type.

Definition—an agonist

An agonist is a drug that has an affinity for a receptor and once bound to that receptor causes a specific response, e.g. morphine which binds to mu (μ) receptors in the CNS depressing the feeling of pain (☐ Action of opioid analgesics).

Definition—an antagonist

An antagonist or receptor-blocker is a drug which has an affinity for a receptor but does not cause a specific response.

- Antagonists reduce the likelihood of other drugs/endogenous ligands binding and therefore further drug/ligand activity is blocked or reduced.
- Competitive antagonists compete with agonists for receptor sites mitigating the action of the agonist by reducing its opportunity for action, e.g. naloxone is used for opioid overdose as it will compete with morphine for μ receptors.
- Non-competitive agonists are receptor blockers which prevent an agonist from having an effect.
- Drug to receptor binding is reversible and a drug action reduces once it has left the receptor site.

Partial agonists can act on receptor sites but their maximal effect is less than a complete agonist.

Interference with ion passages/channels through the cell membrane

An ion is an atom or group of atoms that have lost one or more electrons (cation) or gained one or more electrons (anion).

An ion passage/channel is a selective pore in the cell membrane that allows the movement of ions in and out of the cell.

Drugs which block these channels, such as the calcium channel blocker nifedipine, cause an interference with ion transport and an altered physiological response.

Enzyme inhibition or stimulation

An enzyme is a protein acting as a catalyst in a specific biochemical reaction.
- Some drugs interact with enzymes as their receptors.
- ACE inhibitors and aspirin act in this way. Insulin is destroyed by proteolytic enzymes.

Incorporation into macromolecules

Some drugs are incorporated into macromolecules (larger molecules) and alter the normal functioning of that molecule.

Drugs of this type are used for cancer treatment e.g. 5-fluorouracil which is incorporated into ribonucleic acid (RNA) taking the place of uracil and altering the message carried by the RNA.

Interference with the metabolic processes of microorganisms

Some antibiotics kill the infection-causing microorganism e.g penicillin which disrupts the ability of the bacteria to form cell walls.

Non-specific mechanisms

Chemical alteration of the cellular environment

Some drugs do not alter specific cell function but cause the chemical environment surrounding the cell to alter which changes the normal cellular responses.

Osmotic laxatives and antacids are examples of this type of drug.

Physical alteration of the cellular environment

Drugs in this class alter the physical environment surrounding the cell which cause alterations in the normal cellular responses. Barrier preparations which protect the skin work on this principle.

Pharmacokinetics

The movement of drugs within the body and the way in which the body changes drugs over time. There are four basic processes:
- drug absorption
- drug distribution
- drug metabolism
- drug excretion

Drug absorption

Conveying the drug from the site of administration into the circulatory or lymphatic system.
- Almost all drugs require absorption into the body before they can have any effect.
- The proportion of a drug which has reached the general circulation is termed its bioavailability.
- Drugs which are administered intravenously (IV) are said to have 100% bioavailability.
- Administration by routes other than IV lead to a decrease in bioavailability as some molecules of the drug will be lost during the absorption and distribution processes.
- Drugs administered orally are absorbed from the gastrointestinal (GI) tract, and are carried by the hepatic portal vein to the liver.
- Metabolism of the drug may start in the liver and this is referred to as the first pass effect.

Definition—first pass effect

First pass effect is the removal of a drug by the liver before the drug has had any therapeutic effect.
- First pass effect renders some drugs inactive and necessitates their administration by another route.
- Glyceryl trinitrate (GTN) is an example of a drug which is rendered less active by the first pass effect and is therefore taken by sublingual or transdermal routes.
- 📖 Therapeutic range.

Absorption following oral administration

Most drugs present in the gut in solution (stronger solution) will pass through the cell membrane into the blood stream (weaker solution) by passive diffusion (the concentration gradient). This process will continue until there is an equal concentration on either side of the cell membrane. Passive diffusion is an energy neutral process.

Some lipid soluble drugs require facilitated diffusion in order to cross the cell membrane in combination with a carrier molecule. Facilitated diffusion also requires a concentration gradient and requires no energy expenditure. Some drugs, which resemble substances occurring in the body, are absorbed against the concentration gradient and require carrier molecules and energy to be expended. This is called active transport.

Factors affecting drug absorption from the GI tract
- Gut motility—if motility is increased, less of the drug is absorbed.
- Gastric emptying—if increased, the absorption rate of the drug is increased; if slowed, the absorption rate of the drug is decreased.
- Surface area—rate of drug absorption is greatest in the small intestine as it is lined with villi, which increase the overall surface area.
- Gut pH—this varies along the length of the gut and this changing environment may prevent optimal absorption of a drug in some areas.
- Blood flow—↑ absorption rates in areas with good blood supply (maintaining a good concentration gradient).
- Presence of food and fluid—may increase or decrease drug absorption depending on the drug e.g. absorption of tetracycline is reduced if there are dairy products present in the gut.
- Antacids—these affect the pH and therefore the absorption rates.
- Drug composition—liquid preparations are absorbed more quickly than solid ones, and lipid soluble preparations more quickly than aqueous ones.

Absorption following parenteral administration
- Intradermal drugs diffuse slowly from the injection site into local capillaries.
- Subcutaneous drugs are absorbed more quickly than intradermal.
- Intramuscular (IM) drugs are absorbed faster than intradermal or subcutaneous.

Absorption following topical administration
- Lower rates of absorption than parenteral or oral administration.
- Rate is increased if the skin is broken or an occlusive dressing used.
- Faster absorption if a highly vascular area—e.g. rectum, sublingual.
- Nasal route allows for local as well as systemic absorption.
- Inhalation into the lungs provides extensive absorption.
- Minimal absorption from the ear.
- Absorption from the eye depends on whether the drug is in solution or ointment.

Sometimes the drug is required to stay in place and absorbtion is not required e.g. eczema.
📖 Suitability of formulation.

Drug distribution

The transportation of the drug from the site of administration to the target area. During this process, the molecules of some drugs may be deposited at storage sites and other drugs may be deposited and inactivated.

Factors influencing drug distribution

- Blood flow—drug distribution is faster if the organ has a good blood supply e.g. heart or liver rather than less vascular e.g. bone.
- Plasma protein binding—in circulation drugs may either be bound to a protein, usually albumin, or 'free' and unbound. Only free drug molecules can cause an effect and as free molecules leave the circulation others are released from the protein to which they are bound to re-establish the fraction of those free and those bound.
- Displacement of one bound drug by another—this can have serious consequences i.e. if warfarin is displaced by tolbutamide this may precipitate haemorrhage as there is a greater amount of free warfarin in the circulation or if tolbutamide is displaced by salicylates this may cause hypoglycaemia.
- Placental barrier—permits the passage of poorly lipid soluble drugs from the mother to the fetus but prohibits the passage of lipid soluble preparations.
- Blood–brain barrier—CNS capillaries have a different structure to those elsewhere in the body and this constrains the passage of lipid-insoluble drugs.
- Storage sites—fat tissue acts as a storage facility for lipid-soluble drugs and calcium containing structures such as bones and teeth can accumulate drugs that bind to calcium. Drugs may accumulate in these sites and not be released until after their administration has ceased.

Drug metabolism

The process of modifying or altering the chemical composition of the drug is also called biotransformation.

During this process:
- the pharmacological activity of the drug is removed (but sometimes enhanced first e.g pro-drugs)
- metabolites (products of the drug's metabolism) are produced
- metabolites are more water soluble than the drug itself and this promotes their excretion from the body
- metabolic processes include oxidation, reduction, hydrolysis, and conjugation
- most drug metabolism occurs in the liver, catalysed by hepatic enzymes
- other sites for metabolism are the kidneys, intestinal mucosa, lungs, plasma, and placenta.

Certain drugs, if given repeatedly, are metabolized more rapidly in subsequent doses due to enzyme induction. This requires the drug to be given in larger and larger doses to achieve the same affect as the initial dose. This is sometimes referred to as drug tolerance, although tolerance may also be caused by changes to the drug receptors within the cells.

Factors influencing drug metabolism

- Genetic differences—enzyme systems are genetically determined.
- Age—in older people, first pass metabolism may be reduced or there may be a delayed production and elimination of metabolites resulting in increased bioavailability of the drug. Reduced doses may be indicated for older people.
- In neonates the enzyme systems responsible for conjugation of the drug may be incompletely developed increasing the risk of the toxic effects of the drugs.
- Disease process—any alteration in the body systems caused by a disease process has the potential to alter the metabolism or response to a drug, e.g. liver disease reduces hepatic blood flow which slows the metabolism of a drug leading to an accumulation of the drug and eventually toxicity.
- Mental and emotional factors—confusion, depression, amnesia, stress, and other mental illnesses may reduce a patient's capabilities and motivation which can result in their inability to correctly follow a medication regimen e.g. anorexia and dehydration may already have altered the individual's metabolism.
- Genetic factors—genetic variations lead to differences in metabolic reactions to medication, i.e. patients genetically inheriting the possession of an atypical form of the enzyme pseudocholinesterase have a prolonged paralysis and reaction time when given the muscle relaxant suxamethonium.
- Ethnicity—metabolism of drugs varies from one ethnic group to another. It is also important to remember that different cultures have different health beliefs and practices.

Table 4.1. Some common food or herb and drug interactions [1-5]

Food or herb	Drug	Reaction	Reason
Fruit juice Grapefruit	Simvastatin Atorvastatin	Headache, muscle weakness	Reduced metabolism and elimination
Fruit juice grapefruit	Nifedipine	Hypotension, tachycardia and flushing	
Barbecued meat	Diazepam	The dose will need to be increased to obtain the therapeutic effect	Accelerates the action of enzymes in the gut and liver
St John's Wort	Antidepressants	Mild serotonin syndrome	Inhibits enzymes clearing selective serotonin reuptake inhibitors (SSRIs)
Liquorice	Corticosteroids	Fluid retention, hypertension, hypokalaemia	Decreased renal clearance
100–200g/day of liquorice	Antihypertensives	Fluid retention, hypertension, hypokalaemia	Retention of corticosteroid hormones
Ginko and ginseng	NSAIDs	Bleeding	Interfere with clotting
Garlic, ginko, ginger, feverfew, cranberry juice	Warfarin	Bleeding	Platelet dysfunction
St John's Wort, ginseng, camomile, brewed green tea	Warfarin	Clotting	Drug inactivated
Evening primrose oil	Antipsychotics	Possible increased risk of seizures	Possible additive effect

1 Dresser, G., Bailey, D., Leake, BF., et al. (2000) Fruit Juices inhibit organic anion transporting polypeptide- mediated rug uptake to decrease the oral availability of fexofenadine. *Clinical Pharmacology and Therapeutics,* **71**, 1.

2 Fugh–Berman, A. (2000) Herb-drug interactions. *The Lancet,* **355**, 9198.

3 Karch, A. (200) *Focus on Nursing Pharmacology* (2nd ed). Lippincott Philadelphia.

4 Sorenson, J. (2002). Herb-drug, food-drug, nutrient-drug and drug-drug interactions: mechanisms involved and their medical implications. *The Journal of Alternative and Complementary Medicine,* **8**, 3.

5 Stockley, I. (1999). *Drug interactions* (5th edn). Blackwell Science, Oxford.

Drug excretion

The elimination of drugs and their metabolites from the body. Most drugs and metabolites of drugs are excreted through the kidneys.

Factors affecting the rate of excretion of drugs and metabolites through the kidneys
• Presence of kidney disease
• Altered renal blood flow
• pH of urine
• Concentration of drug in plasma
• Molecular weight of the drug.

Bile
• Some drugs and metabolites are secreted from the liver into the bile and then via the common bile duct to the duodenum.
• Some drugs may be reabsorbed from the terminal ileum and then return to the liver. This is called enterohepatic recycling.
• Enterohepatic recycling may extend the duration of action of the drug.
• Drugs eventually pass to the large intestine and are eliminated in the faeces.

Lungs
Pulmonary excretion accounts for small amounts of alcohol and anaesthetic gases.

Breast milk
Small amounts of a drug may pass from the capillaries surrounding the milk-producing glands and be ingested by a suckling infant who may be unable to metabolize and excrete the drug (📖 Breast feeding).

Perspiration, saliva, and tears
Some lipid soluble drugs may be passively excreted via these routes (some anti-epileptic drugs are secreted in saliva and their levels can be monitored from saliva samples).

Half–life of a drug

The time taken for the concentration of a drug in the plasma to fall by 50%, half its original value.
• Many standard dose calculations are based on this value.
• It allows a dose to be calculated which produces a stable plasma concentration and is below the toxic value and above the minimum effective level.

Loading dose

A dose which is larger than the normal dose and allows a plasma steady state to be reached quickly.

- A maintenance dose is subsequently given
- It is useful to give a loading dose for antibiotic therapy or digoxin.

Therapeutic drug monitoring (TDM)

The term used when regular plasma levels of a drug are taken in order to ensure that a drug with a narrow therapeutic index is used effectively.

- Drugs such as digoxin, lithium, and phenytoin are monitored in this way.
- It is also used as a tool to check patient concordance with a regimen.

Therapeutic index

The therapeutic index is the ratio of a drug's toxic dose to its minimally effective dose (📖 Therapeutic range).

Volume of distribution (Vd)

- The Vd can be calculated from the drug concentration in the bloodstream.
- Drugs are distributed unevenly between various body fluids and tissues according to their physical and chemical properties.
- High lipid solubility allows a drug to cross membranes.
- High tissue protein binding properties leaves less of the drug in the plasma, e.g gentamicin has good water solubility and poor lipid solubility and therefore stays mainly in body fluids and blood.
- A low Vd indicates that the drug is mainly confined to blood and body water as with gentamicin.
- A high Vd indicates the drug has overflowed into the tissues.

Uses of Vd

- If a drug is highly distributed to the tissues the first few doses are not apparent in the blood stream.
- The use of a loading dose (see above) is indicated to enable the dose to be both in the tissue and blood stream.
- This is important if the site of action of the dose is in the tissues, e.g digoxin.
- Vd can be used to help calculate the dose needed to achieve critical plasma concentration.

Prescribing for the extremes of life

Both the very old and very young have problems with excretion and breakdown of drugs ($\square$ Metabolism).

- Healthy neonates (newborns) have a degree of renal and hepatic insufficiency resulting in incomplete metabolism of drugs and raised levels of toxicity. Neonates also have an increased water to fat ratio for the first 28 days after their birth and therefore need higher doses of some drugs e.g. aminoglycosides. It is beyond the scope of this handbook to give guidance on prescribing for the very young and specialist advice is required.
- Healthy older people often have a degree of renal impairment which delays drug excretion through the kidneys, thus increasing the duration of action of a preparation. However, when suffering from an acute illness a further and rapid reduction in renal clearance will exacerbate this process. Liver function may also be impaired resulting in delayed drug metabolism.

$\square$ Prescribing for older people.
$\square$ Prescribing for children.

How to calculate Vd

$$Vd = \frac{X}{Cp}$$

Where X = the total amount of drug in the body
Cp = the plasma concentration of the drug
Vd = the volume of distribution

How to calculate the loading dose

Loading dose (LD) = (Vd) × (Cp)

$\square$ Drug effects.
$\square$ ADRs.

Chapter 5

Potential and unwanted effects

Drug effects

The effect that a drug (or drugs) has on the body:
- can be beneficial
- can be harmful adverse drug effects (ADEs).

Adverse drug reactions (ADRs) and adverse drug interactions (ADIs):
- cause 2–6% of admissions to hospital
- cause 0.24–2.9% deaths of hospital inpatients[1]
- can affect the quality of life
- can be costly
- can copy symptoms of disease
- can affect concordance.

📖 Basic principles of pharmacology.
📖 Adverse drug reactions.

Adverse drug reaction

Definition

A reaction related to the use of a specific drug or drugs which causes harm and/or discomfort beyond its predictable therapeutic effects, and which predictably may cause harm to the patient in the future if given in the smaller or larger dose or in the same dosage and regimen. With any ADR, treatment may warrant prevention of future reactions or alteration of the drug and dosage regimen and possible withdrawal of the product.

Causes

- The drug–pharmacological or physiological actions of a drug (often common and predictable).
- The patient's response to the drug (often rare, idiosyncratic, unavoidable, and unpredictable).
- Prescribing error or inappropriate prescribing.

When making prescribing decisions remember:
- any drug has the potential for adverse drug reactions and interactions (some more than others)
- as part of baseline prescribing assessment when prescribing more than one drug, always consider risk versus benefit for the patient, in partnership with the patient, and with the independent prescriber for supplementary prescribing
- special precautions and contraindications are indicated in the British National Formulary (BNF)[2] see Appendix 1 (BNF) and by the Committee on Safety of Medicines (CSM)
- always document an adverse drug reaction in the patient's notes/computerized records.

Further reading

World Health Organization (1966). *International drug monitoring: the role of the hospital.* WHO, Geneva.

1 Kelly, J. (2000). *Adverse drug effects: A nursing concern.* Whurr, London.
2 British Medical Association and Royal Pharmaceutical Society of Great Britain. *British National Formulary* (latest edn). BMA, London.

Adverse drug reactions (ADRs)

  📖 Basic principles of pharmacology.
  📖 Classification of adverse drug effects and drug interactions.

Drug reactions

- The reaction the body has to a drug.
- Can carry clinical significance and cause a noticeable effect.
- May not be clinically significant.
- Can be beneficial (levodopa/carbidopa in Parkinson's disease).
- Can be harmful (ADR).
- More common in older people as a result in changes in pharmacokinetics and pharmacodynamics, polypharmacy, and polymorbidity.

Classification of frequency of side effects

- *Very common:* > 1 in 10
- *Common:* 1 in 100 to 1 in 10
- *Uncommon:* 1 in 1000 to 1 in 100
- *Rare:* 1 in 10 000 to 1 in 1000
- *Very rare:* < 1 in 10 000[1].

Some patients will experience side effects when they first start to take the drug and these side effects may abate with time. If prescribing drugs with known adverse side effects, but which have been considered to be of benefit to the patient, inform patients of known side effects and urge patient to persevere (e.g. combined contraceptive pill).

Minimizing ADRs

- Identify patients who are taking potentially interacting drugs.
- Only use a drug where there is good indication and where benefit exceeds risk.
- Always ask the if the patient is taking other medications, including drugs and herbal medicines, purchased over the counter.
- Identify high-risk groups, including older people, children, pregnant and breastfeeding women, and patients with polymorbidity or subject to polypharmacy. Only use for these special groups if a full risk/benefit assessment has been completed.
- Always ask about allergy and previous ADRs.
- Use as few concurrent drugs as possible.
- Gradually titrate to greatest therapeutic effect.
- Start with the lowest effective dose and if appropriate reduce dose.

Monitoring adverse drug reactions

Through yellow card reporting of adverse reactions for any drug given to patients in UK to the Medicines and Health Care Products Regulatory Agency (MHRA):

Medicines and Healthcare Products Regulatory Agency (MHRA)
Committee on Safety of Medicines (CSM) Freepost
London SW8 5BR, UK[1]
Online reporting to MHRA at medicines.mhra.gov.uk
Tel: 24-hour freephone (0800 731 6789)

- Report suspected ADRs to any drug, including those self-medicated by the patient, also report reactions to blood products, vaccines, radiographic contrast media, and herbal products.
- Can report drugs of any age.
- Can be used by all prescribers.
- Confidential.
- No blame attached.

The Pharmacovigilance Unit monitors safety of marketed drugs and works with the CSM, advising the government on the licensing of medicines and their safety.

Report

- Black triangle drugs: these are new drugs. The black triangle indicates that their safety profile is being closely monitored ▼.
- Serious reactions with established drugs e.g. those that have been on the market for more than 2 years.
- All ADRs in children.
- All ADRs for complementary and unlicensed medicines.
- Record in patient's notes.

Post marketing surveillance

- Detects risks in a target population after the drug has been marketed.
- Establishes efficacy for the population in general.
- Establishes cost effectiveness.
- Identifies therapeutic benefits which were not previously predicted.
- Interprofessional cooperation between all prescribers, pharmacists, and patients/carers can help to avoid ADRs.

📖 Seven principles of safe prescribing.

Further reading

Grahame-Smith, Aronson, J.K. (2002). *Oxford Textbook of Clinical Pharmacology and Drug Therapy* (3rd edn). Oxford University Press, Oxford.

Kelly, J. (2000). *Adverse drug effects: A nursing concern.* Whurr, London.

Pirmohamed, M., Breckenridge, A.M., Kitleringham, N.R., *et al.* (1998). Adverse drug reactions *BMJ*, **316**, 1295–8.

Adverse drug interactions (ADIs)

Definition
Alteration of the drug's effects by the prior or concurrent administration of another drug (drug–drug interactions) or by food (drug–food interactions)[1]

📖 Basic principles of Pharmacology.

Drug interactions
- The modification of the effect of one drug by the administration of another or with several different drugs.
- Can be beneficial.
- Can be harmful (ADIs).
- May affect normal body processes.
- Effects can be opposing each other or additive (synergistic) effects: the combined effect of two drugs.

📖 Basic principles of pharmacology.
📖 ADRs.
📖 Drug effects.

Types of interactions
- Pharmacokinetic: drug absorption, distribution, metabolism, and excretion.
- Pharmacodynamic: antagonism of one drug at the receptor site changes the effect of the drug.

📖 Basic principles of pharmacology.

Interactions can occur between one drug or group of drugs with another drug or group of drugs:
- during absorption, distribution, metabolism, and excretion
- as a result of competition at the site of action
- they can be additive and potentiate an effect, or antagonistic and block an effect.

Serious interactions can occur as a result of inhibition or induction of metabolic enzymes by one drug or drugs, leading to an increase or decrease in plasma concentrations of another drug or drugs.[2]

A list of likely drug-drug and drug-food interactions can be found in Appendix 1 of the British National Formulary (BNF).[3]

📖 Classification of adverse drug effects and drug interactions.

1 📖 Merck (2006) http://www.merck.com/mrkshared/mmanual/section22/sec22.jsp
2 McGavock, H. (2003). *How drugs work: Basic pharmacology for healthcare professionals.* Radcliffe Medical Press, Oxford.
3 British Medical Association and Royal Pharmaceutical Society of Great Britain. *British National Formulary* (latest edn). BMA, London.

Classification of adverse drug effects and drug interactions[1,2]

Refer to appendix in the latest BNF.

Type A effects: augmented
Aetiology
- Dose related.
- Usually relate to the pharmacology of the drug.
- Are responsible for at least 80% of adverse drug effects.
- Can be of therapeutic benefit.
- Can cause toxicity or decreased therapeutic benefit.
- Can be harmful for the patient.

Actions to prevent/minimize effects
- Take a thorough past and current medical history including past or current drug interactions and allergies.
- Take a thorough history of current medication.
- Ask about any medication purchased over 'or under' the counter.
- Record prescribing actions in shared medical notes and in patient's hand-held records.
- Start with lowest effective dose.
- Reducing the dose may resolve the problem.
- Gradually titrate dose to greatest therapeutic effect.
- Where applicable, administer drug only to required site of action, e.g. inhaled corticosteroids.
- Target drug to treat specific condition, e.g organism-specific antimicrobials.
- Use NPC prescribing pyramid[3] to complete holistic prescribing assessment.

Examples
- Concomitant use of antihypertensives leading to hypotension.
- Concurrent administration of drugs to maximize effects.
- NSAIDs and opioid analgesics for pain control.
- Beta antagonist and diuretic for hypertension.

1 Kelly J (2000) Adverse Drug Effects a Nursing Concern. London. Whurr
2 Rawlins, M.D. and Thompson, J.W. (1977) Pathogenesis of adverse drug reactions. In: *Textbook of adverse drug reactions*, ed. D.M. Davies. Oxford University Press, Oxford.
3 National Prescribing Centre (1999). *Signposts for prescribing nurses – general principles of good prescribing*. National Prescribing Centre Liverpool.

Type B effects: bizarre

Aetiology
- Rare.
- Unpredictable.
- Unrelated to dose.
- Idiosyncratic.
- Hard to prevent in the first instance.
- Relatively high morbidity and mortality.

Actions to prevent/minimize effects
- As for type A effects.
- Ask about family history of allergies/reactions.
- Ask about patient's history of allergies.
- Ask about drugs purchased over and 'under the counter'.

Examples
- Anaphylactic immunological reaction to a specific antibiotic.
- Statins myositis, myalgia, myopathy.

Type C: chronic effects

Aetiology
- Result from long-term drug usage.
- Usually associated with treatment for chronic disease.

Actions to prevent/minimize effects
As for Type A and Type B effects.

Examples
- Tolerance to nicotine.
- Osteoporosis with steroids.

Type D: delayed effects

Aetiology
Can occur many years after therapy has stopped.

Actions to prevent/minimize effects
As above and:
- monitoring, audit.
- clinical research.
- longitudinal post-marketing surveillance.

Examples
Stilboestrol and vaginal cancer.

Type E: end of use effects
Aetiology
- Occur as a result of abrupt cessation of some therapies, e.g. systemic anabolic steroids.
- Withdrawal from some antidepressants.

Type F: effect failure
Aetiology
Failure of drug to achieve therapeutic effect.

Actions to prevent/minimize effects
Give adequate information and advice as to how to take, when to take, and precautionary measures.

Examples
Inadequate dose of contraceptive when used with rifampicine.

Further reading
McGavock, H. (2003). *How Drugs Work: Basic Pharmacology For Healthcare Professionals*. Radcliffe Medical Press Oxford.
Stockley, I. H. (ed.) (2005). *Stockeley's Drug Interactions*. Pharmaceutical Press, London.

Therapeutic range/index

There is a range within which plasma concentrations will be related to therapeutic effect. Concentrations below this range have little therapeutic effect. Toxicity is related to increasing concentration and may occur within the therapeutic range of a drug or in concentrations above this range. Special care needs to be taken with certain drugs that have a narrow therapeutic range: where the plasma concentration is higher than the therapeutic range, severe adverse drug reactions can occur.

Drugs with a narrow therapeutic range/index

- Methotrexate
- Digoxin
- Warfarin
- Lithium
- Theophylline
- Phenytoin
- Valproate.

Plasma protein binding

Most drugs bind to plasma protein and are transported around the body in this way. A drug which is bound to plasma protein is not available to the body for use. It is the free drug which exerts its effect. The concentration of the free drug rises when the drug is displaced from the plasma protein. Some drugs, such as phenytoin and other antiepileptic drugs can be highly plasma protein bound (>90%). If phenytoin is displaced from its plasma protein binding by other drugs, an increase in plasma concentration of phenytoin will occur without a change in total concentration. Toxicity can occur with rapid displacement.

Steady state

This is a constant state of balance between the metabolism and elimination of a drug from the body and the absorption of a drug into the body to replace that which is metabolized and eliminated.

Half-life and toxicity

Half-life

- This is the time taken for the plasma concentration of a drug to fall by half.
- It is important to understand half-life when considering the potential toxic effects of drugs on the body.
- It is used to predict the rate of accumulation of a drug in the body.
- It can be used to predict the length of time a drug takes to be eliminated from the body.
- It takes approximately 5 half-lives to achieve steady state and as long again for a drug to be eliminated from the body.

Some drugs have a very long half-life, e.g. such as digoxin (40 hrs).

Toxicity
- This refers to any adverse reaction by the body to the administration of drugs for therapeutic purposes, regardless of dosage or amount.
- Displacement of digoxin from plasma protein can, and does, lead to toxicity.
- Digoxin would take 160–200 hrs to leave the body; this can cause problems in states of toxicity.

📖 Basic principles of pharmacology.

Special precautions

Drugs of bioequivalence act on the body with the same strength and similar bioavailability at the same dosage, although they may be different formulations or chemical compounds. When prescribing most drugs the prescriber is encouraged to use the non-proprietary title (name) of the drug as this supports the prescribing of any suitable product of bioequivalence; so if one drug is not available, another brand can be dispensed. However, it is important to note that in some drugs, it is important to prescribe by brand name rather than by generic name.

📕 Drug effects.
📕 Adverse drug reactions (ADRs).

Managing ADEs (in the event of toxicity)
- If the patient is having difficulty breathing or is not breathing maintain airway.
- Take a history of events.
- Keep evidence.
- Reduce or stop dose.
- Assess vital signs.

Review of prescribing web sites

🖳 *Pharmaceutical Journal: www.pharmj.com*

This is the electronic version of the *Pharmaceutical Journal*. Subscription is free and it provides an excellent source of evidence-based information, including continuing professional development (CPD) with a pharmacist-based slant. The web site links to Clinical Evidence, BMJ publishing group. This publication has up-to-date reviews of clinical evidence related to prescribing. It is useful for systematic reviews of up-to-date randomized control trials and clinical comparison of drugs and their clinical application.

🖳 *Prodigy Knowledge: www.prodigy.nhs.uk*

This site provides patient, nurse, and doctor information for a wide range of disease management. The site provides brief updates which inform practice. The site provides information leaflets with patient-friendly diagrams, as well as details of self-help groups, patient groups, and similar organizations.

🖳 *Association of the British Pharmaceutical Industry: www.abpi.org.uk*

This site contains useful information pertaining to the drug industry, its code of conduct and vital statistics. The site includes some patient information produced by drug companies and summaries of product characteristics.

🖳 *Prescriber/escriber: www.am-publishing.co.uk/prescriber.html*

The online electronic journal *Prescriber* covers peer-reviewed articles relating to primary care, therapeutics, and prescribing-related issues. Good for research articles about pharmacology, pharmacokinetics, and pharmacodynamics. The site links to NICE guidelines and the National Service Frameworks (NSFs) and also has medical humour.

🖳 *National Prescribing Centre (NPC): www.npc.co.uk*

Links to sites related to clinical governance, knowledge and skills framework, standards, and competencies related to prescribing. This site provides authoritative and up-to-date information on all aspects of medical and non-medical prescribing. The site also produces MeReC bulletins.

🖳 *Medicines and Health Care Regulatory Agency: www.mhra.gov.uk.*

This excellent site is devoted to protecting the public, maintaining, and regulating standards for the pharmaceutical industry, and prescribing. It provides comprehensive information on how products are licensed and information related to prescribing and public health.

🖳 *National electronic Library for Health (NeLH): www.nelh.nhs.uk*

Links to all major academic and information sites for prescribing, including BNF, Cochrane data base, Clinical Evidence, Drugs and Therapeutics Bulletin.

▣ *Scottish Intercollegiate Guidelines Network (SIGN):* *www.sign.ac.uk*
This site is the Scottish equivalent of NICE. Links with NICE, to work in partnership to provide evidence-based guidelines for standardized treatment for disease management. Good, reliable source of evidence-based information.

▣ *UKMIPG-UK Medicines Information Pharmacists Group:*
www.ukmi.nhs.uk
This site is a source of up-to-date online information for pharmacists working in primary care. Useful links to National Electronic Library for Medicine www.nlm.nih.gov/databases and specialist advice services. Interesting link to www.quackwatch.com

▣ *Medicines:* *www.medicines.org.uk*
Provides a summary of product characteristics for drugs and a search engine for information regarding specific medicines.

▣ *Free Medical Journals.com:* *www.freemedicaljournals.com*
This site provides access to useful free online journals.

▣ *Chemist and Druggist:* *www.dotpharmacy.com*
Useful for self-testing for continuing professional development (CPD).

▣ *Drug and Therapeutics Bulletin:* *www.which.net/health/dtb*
Up-to-date information regarding common drugs.

▣ *Hospital Pharmacist:* *www.pharmj.com/backissues.html*
Has lots of information about medicines management. Good access to free electronic journals related to prescribing. Useful updates from *Pharmaceutical Journal* online.

▣ *Bandolier:* *www.jr2.ox.ac.uk/bandolier*
Rich source for evidence-based pharmacology and prescribing.

▣ *British Medical Journal (BMJ):* *www.bmj.com*
Access to evidence-based medicine, news, and reviews.

▣ *British National Formulary:* *www.bnf.org/*
This site provides an online up-to-date BNF if you subscribe to the site. It has lots of links to useful sites related to prescribing.

Where to get up-to-date information

See also 📖 Using the BNF and 📖 Review of prescribing web sites.

National guidelines

The National Institute for Health and Clinical Excellence (NICE) provides up-to-date technology appraisals, which are nationally recognized guidelines that adhere to best clinical evidence and which recommend best practice and cost-effective prescribing. Technology appraisals are updated every 5 years.

Nationally recognized guidelines are also produced by:
- 🖳 the British Thoracic society (BTS): www.brit.thoracic.org.uk
- 🖳 the British Hypertensive Society (BHS): www.bhs.org.uk
- 🖳 the British Diabetic Association (BDA): www.diabetes.org.uk
- 🖳 the British Heart Foundation (BHF): www.bhft.org.uk
- 🖳 and Scottish Intercollegiate Guidelines Network (SIGN): www.sign.ac.uk

Prodigy Knowledge (www.prodigy.nhs.uk) provides a nationally recognized knowledge source for nurse independent and supplementary prescribers in primary and secondary care.

Local guidelines

Locally produced NHS formularies provide evidence-based guidelines, and protocols for prescribing medications and appliances, they also advise on locally accepted practice and safe and cost-effective prescribing.

Guidelines are exactly what they say, and in supplementary prescribing, in agreement with the independent prescriber and the patient, can be tailored to meet the needs of the individual patient. However, whenever possible, it is best practice for the nurse prescriber who is working for the NHS to follow the guidelines as indicated both nationally and within the local NHS formulary.

PACT data

PACT (prescribing analysis and cost) and SPA (Scottish prescribing analysis) are available as audit reports of practitioners prescribing on a quarterly (3 monthly) basis. This data provides comparisons between local and national prescribing patterns and can be broken down to indicate individual prescribing patterns.
📖 Audit.
📖 Prescription analysis and cost (PACT).

The Drug Tariff

The Drug Tariff is produced monthly as a joint compilation between the Department of Health and the Prescription Pricing Authority[1] (now renamed the Business Services Authority).

---

1 Department of Health. *Drug Tariff* (latest version). HMSO, London. 🖳 Available at www.ppu.org.uk

Useful information contained in the drug tariff:
- the basic price of named drugs, appliances, and chemical reagents
- endorsements including pack sizes
- whether the prescription is in phamacopoeial or generic form
- brand name and name of manufacturer or wholesaler from whom the drug was purchased
- quantity supplied (if at variance with quantity ordered)
- pharmacists' professional payments fees
- commonly used pack sizes
- advice on domiciliary oxygen service
- advice to care homes
- borderline substances
- the dental prescribing formulary
- the district nurse and health visitor prescribers' formulary
- the nurse prescribers' extended formulary
- drugs and other substances not to be prescribed under the NHS pharmaceutical services (blacklisted drugs)
- drugs to be prescribed in certain circumstances under the NHS pharmaceutical services.

Holistic assessment

In contrast to the medical model of assessment which seeks to identify a problem from symptoms, investigations, and physical examination and then make a curative response, an holistic nursing assessment takes into account the physical, emotional, psychological, and environmental or social aspects of the symptoms and feelings presented by the patient, their family, or carers. Notions of well-being, quality of life, and the values and aspirations of the individual are also considered.

The non-reductive, holistic account of health derives from exploration of what it is to be a person and the acceptance that persons are partly defined by their aspirations and goals and this extends to their notions of illness and wellbeing.

There is a fundamental difference between the biomedical model which decides if a person is ill by examination and requires no input from the patient and the holistic account of ill health which includes the patients own view of the matter.

Helen Close[1] suggests the nurse prescriber may find it useful to adapt a seven point holistic assessment model from Twycross and Black[2] originally for use in the treatment of nausea and vomiting but applicable to more general use:

1. **Evaluation of the history given by the patient**
- Time and onset of symptoms.
- Physical, emotional, and social effects of the symptoms.
- Past and current medical history, current prescribed medication, including over the counter (OTC) and 'borrowed medication', and any known allergies.
- Any red flag symptoms e.g. bleeding, obstruction?
2. **Record the severity of the symptoms**
- How often are they experienced?
- Does the patient regard the symptoms as serious?
3. **Correct reversible causes**
- Before treating the symptoms identify any causes which can be eliminated.
4. **Non-drug treatments**
- Are there actions which may be taken to avoid the symptoms?
5. **If needed prescribe and start a drug treatment**
- Move to 5 only when 3 and 4 of the guidelines have failed to give relief of the symptoms.
6. **Check route of administration**
- Optimize effect of treatment by using the most suitable route of administration, e.g a non-oral route if vomiting prevents absorption.
7. **Re-evaluate**
- If there are no improvements in symptoms recommence at 1 and reconsider.
- Clinical or physical examination.
- History taking.
- Using models of consultation for prescribing.
- Concordance.

1 Close, H. (2003). Nausea and vomiting in terminally ill patients: towards a holistic approach. *Nurse Prescribing* **1**, 1.
2 Twycross, R., Black, I. (1998). Nausea and vomiting in advanced cancer care. *European Journal of Palliative Care*, **5** (2), 39–45. ▣ http://www.npc.co.uk/nurse_prescribing/

Concordance

What is concordance?

An informed partnership agreement which is negotiated between the prescriber and the patient.

Holistic assessment and prescribing concordance

An holistic assessment will support concordance and promote harmony.

📖 Holistic assessment.

To establish concordance

Respect the patient

- Involve the patient as an active partner, work in collaboration with the patient to gain a negotiated agreement as to how to proceed.
- Give the appropriate amount and type of information to the patient, at the right place, and at the right time to meet patient needs and appropriate to their level of understanding.
- Make the consultation patient-specific.
- Facilitate patient options and choice.
- Listen to and respect the health beliefs of the patient.
- Use consultation style to break the information into smaller pieces and to check that the patient understands.
- Explain the mode of action of the drug to the patient.
- Tell the patient what to expect.
- Consider and respect the patient's lifestyle, culture, and ethnic background.
- Consider disability, language barriers, and learning disabilities.
- Take the patient's concerns seriously.
- Allow the patient to disagree and take a suboptimal treatment or no treatment.

Communicate

- Speak the patient's language.
- Avoid medical jargon.
- Communicate decisions verbally and in writing.
- Signpost information into a logical sequence.
- Summarize.
- Use patient information leaflets.
- Use pictures/diagrams.
- Look at the patient when talking and listening, not at the computer.
- Observe patient's body language.
- Explain medical tests/terms.

Mutual decision making

- Involves a dialogue between self and the patient.
- What does the patient want?
- What does he or she think/feel?
- Draw up an agreed plan.
- Discuss choices and limitations of choice.
- Consider the options, benefits to the patient, drawbacks to therapy, limitations of agreement.
- Can agree to disagree.

Concordance should be empowering for the patient.

Ask
- What is the patient's initial knowledge base?
- What else do they want/need to know?
- What do they already understand?
- What don't they understand?

Contract with patient, give clear instructions
- Explain how to seek help (safety netting).
- Is the patient happy with the plan?
- Does he/she know what to do?
- When does the plan start?
- 📖 Communication.

Aids to concordance
- Large print leaflets
- Audio and audio visual tapes
- Braille
- Language interpreters
- NHS direct.

Causes of non-concordance
- Lack of patient understanding.
- Lack of patient participation.
- Lack of patient empowerment.
- Unwanted/unpleasant side effects.
- Medication taken over a long period, e.g. chronic disease.
- Cost of medication to patient.
- 📖 Seven principles of safe prescribing.

Further reading
🖳 Medicine's partnership: www.concordance.org
Anon. (2003). News feature. Time to mobilise expert patients' skills. *Pharmaceutical Journal,* **270**, 743–4.

Safe prescribing

Safe prescribing

Accountability

- Document all prescribing decisions and actions.
- Prescribe within the legal framework for nurse independent prescribing and supplementary prescribing.
- Understand that you are legally responsible for prescriptions you write.
- Adhere to Trust policy.
- Do no harm to the patient.
- Adhere to code of conduct.[1]
- Keep up to date with prescribing competencies.[2]
- Only prescribe within your competency area.
- Be aware that you are accountable when you delegate to others.[3]
- Understand the potential for drug abuse and misuse.
- Keep good records.
- Maintain good lines of communication.

Principles

- Follow the principles of prescribing as set out by the National Prescribing Centre.[2]
- Use the prescribing pyramid as a model for prescribing.
- Work as part of a team.
- Understand the pressures that will be placed on you as a prescriber.
- 📖 Seven principles of safe prescribing.

Practice

Practicing legally

- Nurse Independent Prescribers can prescribe licensed drugs from anywhere in the British National Formulary (BNF) providing they are clinically competent to do so.
- As a V100 mode one or mode two prescriber prescribe only from the Community Practitioners' Formulary (CPF).
- As a supplementary prescriber, work in partnership with an independent doctor prescriber and the patient/carer. Give the patient a copy of his or her CMP.
- Always consult the formulary prior to prescribing.

📖 The legal differences between prescribing, administration, and dispensing.
📖 Prescribing and the law.

The practice of assessment

- Only prescribe if you have seen the patient.
- Complete an holistic assessment.
- Follow a structured model of assessment.
- Consider the patient's past medical history.

---

1 Nursing and Midwifery Council (2004). *NMC code of professional conduct: standards for conduct, performance and ethics.* NMC, London.
2 NPC (1999). Signposts for prescribing. *Prescribing Nurse Bulletin* 1(1).
3 Nursing and Midwifery Council (2004). *Guidance for the administration of medicines.* NMC, London.

- Ask about the patient's current health status.
- Take a thorough medication history. Ask about other medication bought over the counter, including herbal remedies.
- Ask about allergies.

The practice of concordance

- Always consider side effects, cautions, contraindications, interactions. Inform the patient of potential side effects, how to take, when to take, how often, dose, what to do if having a reaction.
- Explain the rationale for prescribing to the patient.
- Gain full and informed consent.

📖 Holistic assessment.
📖 Concordance.

Practice safely

- Check that the patient can read the label on the medication.
- Explain how to obtain medicines.
- Advise the patient to keep medicines out of reach of children and animals.
- Advise the patient not to share their medication with others.
- Be aware of the public health implications of your prescribing.

Further reading

Courtney, M. and Butler, M. (2002). *Essential nurse prescribing*. Greenwich Medical Media, London.
Nursing and Midwifery Council (2006). Standards of Nursing and Proficiency for Nurse and Midwife Prescribers. NMC, London.

Responsibility

Responsibility and safety
- Have a clear rationale for prescribing.
- Consider alternatives to prescribing.
- Have a sound knowledge of the therapeutics of any medication you prescribe.
- Give written information to the patient.
- Consider patients who may have special needs.
- Gain concordance between the patient and prescriber.
- Be aware of the needs of patients for whom English is not their first language.
- Prescribe with caution for people from special groups, e.g. renal and hepatic disorders, children, older people, pregnancy, and breastfeeding.
- Review the patient on a regular basis.
- Maintain awareness of limitations of and changes to formularies.
- Be aware of your own limitations in practice.
- Maintain contemporaneous shared record keeping.
- Clear communication with other professionals who are involved in the patient's prescribing journey.
- Report adverse drug reactions, using the yellow card scheme.
- Recognize and analyse critical incidents.
- Understand the requirements of clinical governance.
- Keep up to date with new information.

Responsibility and continuing professional development
- Maintain continuing professional development (CPD).
- Keep your prescribing portfolio up to date.
- Network with other prescribers.
- Develop leadership skills.
- Understand the roles of others.
- Perform audit.
- Share good practice.

📖 Nursing and Midwifery Council (NMC) Code of Professional Conduct: Standards of Conduct, performance, and ethics.

Remember to record: failure to record actions is unsafe practice and constitutes negligence.

📖 Record keeping.

Seven principles of safe prescribing

Prescribing a product or medicine is a complex process which involves far more than writing a prescription and has considerable impact on the patient, colleagues, and the NHS in general. The National Prescribing Centre have a model: the prescribing pyramid which gives a useful framework for prescribing considerations:

The prescribing pyramid

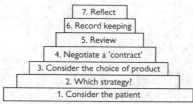

Diagram reproduced with kind permission of the *National Prescribing Centre* from *Nurse Prescribing Bulletin* (1999). Vol 1, No.1. NPC Liverpool

1. Examine the holistic needs of the patient

- Is a prescription really necessary?
- A thorough needs assessment may show that a non-drug therapy is indicated.
- A full medical and social history should be taken, along with an holistic assessment (📖 Holistic assessment), before prescribing.
- The mnemonic 2-WHAM[1] may prove a helpful aide-memoire:
  - **W** Who is it for?
  - **W** What are the symptoms?
  - **H** How long have the symptoms been present?
  - **A** Any action taken so far?
  - **M** Any other medication taken?

When taking a drug history include:
- any prescribed items
- OTC medications
- home remedies (home-made medicines handed down over generations, i.e. an infusion of the plant feverfew for migraine)
- alternative therapies such as homeopathic and herbal remedies
- any prescribed items 'borrowed' from another person
- any known allergies.

---

1 Hayes, A. (1997). Sale of medications in pharmacies: Protocols. Where now? *Pharmaceutical Journal*, **259**, 60–8.
2 Henry, J. (ed.) (1992). *Guide to Medicines and Drugs*. BMA/Dorling Kinsley, London.

2. Consider the appropriate strategy

- Is the diagnosis established?
- Is a GP referral indicated?
- Is a prescription needed at all?
- Is patient expectation a factor in your decision?
- A prescription should only be given when it is genuinely needed. Patients may want prescriptions for reasons other than treatment, for example:
  - to legitimize the sick role
  - to gain attention
  - because a friend had recommended it
  - because a family member or friend would like the product.

3. Consider the product of choice

The use of the mnemonic EASE may be helpful:

E	How effective is the product?
A	Is it appropriate?
S	How safe is it?
E	Is the prescription cost effective?

- To ensure that the product is appropriate, familiarize yourself with the relevant section of the formulary.
- Critically appraise the evidence to assess a product's effectiveness.
- Check the BNF for any ADRs, contraindications, special precautions, or drug interactions.
- Consider dose, formulation, and the duration of treatment with regards to the individual patient.
- Does the patient fall within a particular group requiring specialist knowledge and consideration, e.g. the extremes of life?

📖 Cost effective prescribing.
📖 Adverse drug reactions (ADRs).

4. Negotiating a contract

Shared decision-making between the patient and health-care professional is known as concordance.

- The patient has a central role in the decision-making process.
- The patient needs to understand:
  - what the prescription is for
  - how long it will take to work
  - how to take the product
  - how long to take it for
  - at what dose to take it
  - any possible side effects
  - how and who to contact if the patient has concerns.

📖 Concordance.

5. Reviewing the patient

Regular review will determine whether the prescribed item(s) are effective, safe, and acceptable.

6. Keeping records

The NMC have guidelines regarding record keeping.

📖 Record keeping.

7. Reflecting on your prescribing

Reviewing and reflecting on prescribing decisions will help improve your practice and knowledge base.

📖 Repeat prescriptions.
📖 History and policy.
📖 Concordance.
📖 Safe prescribing.

NB for any given therapeutic intervention, the potential benefits of the intervention must be balanced against safety concerns.

Consideration of product choice

Generic prescribing

- The CPF directs all prescribers to use the generic name of a product when prescribing, rather than the brand name.
- Since 1997 wound care products and appliances can be prescribed by brand name as it was proving very time consuming and confusing to refer to 'vapour permeable adhesive film dressing' for instance when 'OP site®' or 'Tegaderm®' was required.
- Brand names are those given to a particular version of a product by an individual manufacturer.
- Some products are only marketed by one manufacturer however the generic name should still be used when prescribing.
- Other products are only produced in the generic forms.
- Patients should be told that items will be prescribed generically and that although the packaging may differ the content is the same as they have had before; e.g. Canestan cream® pack differs from the clotrimazole pack, although the product is the same.
- Conversely a branded product may be dispensed in place of the generic one prescribed if the branded product is cheaper. PACT data will still record the prescriber as having prescribing generically. www.ePACT.net
- Patients may be reassured that both branded and generic items conform to the licensing requirements of the Medicines Control Agency and are equally safe.
- Products imported from the EU may prove to be less expensive resulting in the patient receiving a product with packaging not in English. Reassurance may be given that the same licensing standards apply and instructions in English are included in the package.
- Since 2000 the free market for the supply and sale of generic products has been regulated by the DoH, which imposes a maximum price.

Some patients need to be kept on branded antiepileptic and lithium products.

📖 Using the BNF

Suitability for formulation

Suitability of formulation

Definition

- The formulation of a medicine refers to its chemical and physical composition.
- This includes both the chemical composition of the active ingredients and those of the excipients which stabilize the active ingredients or modify their release.

It is important to select the appropriate formulation to suit the desired therapeutic outcome and the physical condition, abilities, and psychological inclination of your patient.

Formulations may be:

- Tablets (including dispersible and dissolvable)
- Liquid
- Gums and lozenges
- Patches
- Topical — creams, lotions, emollients, patches etc.
- Rectal
- Parenteral — IV, IM, ID, SC, IT
- Mouthwashes
- Gargles
- Paint/varnish
- For inhalation
- Drops — eye, ear, and nasal.

Considerations include:

Excipients

- May be responsible for some ADRs, for example some penicillins and warfarin contain sodium as do some indigestion remedies and analgesics. Patients with incipient heart failure who take any of these may find the sodium content sufficient to precipitate fluid retention and breathlessness.
- Excipients may vary from one branded product to another and this could have an effect on the bioavailability of the active ingredients. For example with some antiepileptic and lithium preparations if a patient is stable, changing from one branded product to another or to a generic product can result in loss of control of the patient's condition.
- Oral preparations that do not contain fructose, sucrose, or glucose are described as 'sugar free' as are those containing hydrogenated glucose syrup, mannitol, malitol, sorbitol, or xylitol as there is evidence that these do not cause dental caries. This is an important consideration when prescribing for children.

Oral medications

- Tablets and capsules should be swallowed with a glass of water and the patient sitting erect and remaining so for the following 30 mins. This is in order to prevent prolonged contact between a potentially corrosive substance, the medication (bisulphates, aspirin, iron and potassium salts), and the lining of the mouth and oesophagus.

- When prescribing an oral preparation it is important to be aware of potential interactions between drugs, food, and herbs.
- Not only can food affect a drug's bioavailability and alter the therapeutic outcome but drugs can have an adverse impact on a patient's nutritional status.
- **Foods and herbs** may also counteract the action of a drug e.g. fexo fenadine (non-sedating antihistamine) loses effect if taken with orange, apple, or grapefruit juice. Cyclosporine is inactivated by St John's Wort and the metabolism of warfarin is inhibited by grapefruit Juice.
- Drugs and food may bind together leading to their retention in the intestine, e.g. digoxin.
- Administration with food can be beneficial for some preparations e.g. nifedipine as it prevents a sudden onset of action of the drug.
- Some drugs e.g. bisulphates or tetracycline will not be absorbed if given with food.
- **The timing** of administration of enteral or oral medication is impera- tive e.g. iron relies on gastric acidity in order to be absorbed and this may be too low if administered between meals in older people, those with HIV/AIDS and also those taking antacids and H2-receptor agonists.
- Conversely ampicillin and some antivirals for HIV/AIDS, (didanosine, indinvir) are destroyed by stomach acid and therefore should not be taken within 2 hours of meals or enteral feeds.
- **Changing** from a tablet to a liquid preparation of the same medication often requires a reduction of dose.

📕 Where to get up to date information.
📕 Basic principles.
See also the relevant section of the latest version of the BNF.

How to write a prescription

- Nurses can only prescribe within their area of competency.
- Nurses can only prescribe for a patient whom they have assessed.
- They must use the prescription pad which has been issued to them.
- Repeat prescriptions may only be issued under DoH guidelines.
- Repeat prescriptions.

Writing a prescription

- Always use indelible ink, preferably black unless directed otherwise.
- Write legibly.
- Date the prescription.
- State the full name and address of the patient for whom you are prescribing.
- Sign the prescription.
- It is preferable to include the age and date of birth of the patient.
- It is a legal requirement to state the age for a child under 12 years when prescribing a POM.
- The BNF recommends avoidance of the unnecessary use of a decimal point e.g. 3mg not 3.0mg.
- Quantities of 1 gm or more should be written as 1g etc., and quantities of less than 1 gm should be written as 500mg not 0.5 g.
- If the decimal point is unavoidable a zero should be put in front e.g. 0.5ml not .5ml.
- The decimal point may be used when expressing a range i.e. 0.5 to 1g.
- Units, micrograms, and nanograms should not be abbreviated.
- Use the term millilitre (ml or mL) not cubic centimetre cc or cm³.

Details to include:

The name, form, and strength of the item to be dispensed

- Use the generic name except for appliances and dressings.
- Give the dose and frequency of the dose.
- Give full directions on how to use the items.
- Specify the quantity to be supplied — enough to meet the patient's needs but avoiding waste.

Computer generated prescription

- The computer generated prescription must have the date of issue, the patient's second name, forename(s) as initials, and their address printed on it.
- It may print their title and date of birth.
- The age of children under 12 years and adults over 60 must be printed in the box available.
- The age of children less than 5 years should be printed in years and months.
- The prescribers name, surgery address, telephone contact number, forename(s), and reference number should be included.

See latest version BNF for more guidance.

	Age Two	Name (including first names) and address	
	D.o.B 21/5/97	Joanna Bloggs 14 Any Road Fulchester Northshire XS34 4LP	**1. Patient details:** • Full name (surname and first name) • Full address • Age and date of birth
Pharmacy Stamp			

Dispenser's Endorsement	Number of days' treatment N.B. ensure dose is stated		NP		Pricing *Office*

Pack and Quantity	Paracetamol sugar free oral suspension, 120 mg/5ml One 5ml teaspoon to be taken every four to six hours, as required to relieve pain. Max. 4 doses in 24 hours. Supply 100ml Aqueous cream Apply to the affected areas four times a day and use to wash instead of soap. Supply 500g	**2. Details of the item(s) to be supplied:** (a) **Name, form,** and **strength** of the item(s): • Use **generic** name, except for dressings and appliances • Do not use abbreviations (b) **Dose** and **frequency** of dose (c) Directions of how to use the item(s) • Always write **full** directions in English • Do not use abbreviations (d) Quantity to be supplied • Specify and appropriate amount to meet the patient's need while avoiding waste • Generally this should be for no more than one calendar month • Where possible prescribe the pack size specified in the NPF under each preparation – do not use the term 'OP' • Consider patient packs/special containers where appropriate

Signature of Nurse		Date	**3. Signature** of prescriber and date.

For *Dispenser* No. of Presens on form [ ]	Please complete patient's Practice details PATIENTS PRACTICE CODE .... NURSE CONTACT TEL. NO.	**4. Practice Code** – Code for the practice where the patient is registered. **5. Nurse's contact telephone number** The pharmacist must be able to contact the nurse if there is a problem with the prescription.

NHS

Safekeeping of your prescription pad

- Treat your prescription pad with the same care as you would your cheque book.
- Care must be taken to ensure security for the delivery, storage, and use of your prescription pad.
- Some nurses will only take a few prescriptions out with them at a time rather than risk losing the whole pad.
- Prescription pads should be kept in a locked and secure place when not in use.
- It is helpful to record serial numbers of prescriptions as you receive them, and lock away any not yet in use.
- Never leave the prescription pad unattended or visible in the car.
- Never pre-sign a blank prescription form.
- Know and follow your local procedures for lost or stolen pads and scripts (see the box opposite).
- Most areas have a named person to contact who may, as part of their responsibilities, contact the police for you. You are advised to notify local pharmacists and may be requested to complete future prescriptions in a distinctively coloured ink to enable detection of any forgeries.

When not to prescribe

- Do not prsescribe if there is no genuine need.
- Always consider alternatives to a prescription, e.g. in constipation in older people:
  - Are they having sufficient fibre or fluids in their diet?
  - Do they take any exercise?
  - Are they taking another medicine which causes constipation and could be avoided?
  - What is their normal bowel habit?

Why do patients want prescriptions?

- This is a complex issue which requires careful consideration, and treatment of their symptoms is only one possible answer.
- Other reasons why patients may want prescriptions include:
  - to legitimize the sick role
  - to gain attention
  - because a friend had recommended it
  - because a family member or friend would like the product.
- In addition, some patients may wish to sell the product prescribed.

Local procedure for reporting lost or stolen prescription pads

Local procedure:

Name of person to contact:

Telephone/email contact address:

Review

Repeat prescriptions

Approximately 75% of prescriptions are dispensed as repeat prescriptions.[1]

Guidance on repeat prescribing issued by the NHS Executive in 1997 advises that 'no more than 6 repeat prescriptions should be made, or 6 months should elapse, whichever is less, without reassessing the patient's needs'.[2]

The NPC issued the first service improvement guide (SIG) focusing on repeat prescriptions in 2005, which can be accessed from http://www.npc.co.uk

Luker and Austin[3] conducted a review of repeat prescriptions at two of the NP pilot sites and found that many patients were receiving repeat prescriptions of items in the CPF, which had originally been prescribed by doctors. Many of the products were no longer indicated and considerable savings were realized.

It is therefore important to have a system in place which identifies products which a nurse would not usually wish to repeatedly prescribe and it is recommended that 'nurses should be mindful of any protocols already in place'.[2]

Good practice for repeat prescriptions systems
- Written explanation of the process for repeat prescriptions for the patient or their carer.
- Designated personnel with responsibility to ensure the patient recall and regular medication review does take place.
- Agreed policy with the practice on the length of medication supply on a repeat prescription.
- Authorization check made every time a repeat prescription is signed.
- Practice staff to be given training on elements of good practice with regards to patient concordance.
- Records kept up to date.

📖 Seven principles of safe prescribing.
📖 Suitability of formulation.

Adapted from:
Keele University. Department of Medicines Management (2000) *Seizing the opportunities. Report of the Walsall GP/Practice Pharmacy project in DoH Medicines and Older people.*

1 Anon (2003). Repeat dispensing products due to take off in Scotland. *Prescribing and Medicines Management* **1** Jan/Feb 2003.
2 NHS Executive HQ (1997). *Nurse Prescribing Guidance* (April). NHS Executive, Leeds.
3 Luker, K. Austin, L. (1997). Nurse prescribing: study findings and GPs views, *Prescriber*, **8** 31–4.

Format of a detailed medication review

Reviews covering the following core areas may take place in the surgery, an older person's home, or day care facility. They may involve the patient, family members, and/or carers, and should include an explanation of the review's purpose and reasons why it is important.

The review should include:

- a listing of all medicines being taken including:
  - prescribed medicines
  - OTC products
  - herbal medicines
  - homeopathic remedies
  - medicines shared with others
  - homely remedies
  - supplements
- Comparison of the list of medicines used with those prescribed.
- The patient's/carer's perception of the purpose of medicines taken including any misconceptions. A Danish study[1], showed 40% of older people did not know the purpose of their medication.
- The patient's/carer's perception of the frequency, amount and method of taking the medicines including any misconceptions
- Use of the 'prescribing appropriateness indicators'[2] e.g. the indication of the use of the drug in the BNF.
- Any side effects noted including social side effects which restrict people's lives.
- Review of any monitoring tests e.g. HbA1c for diabetes. International Normalized Ratio (INR) for patients taking anticoagulants.
- 📖 Holistic assessment

Types of questions which might be asked of a patient or carer during a medicines review

- How long have you been taking/using this medicine/product?
- Is the medicine in its original container?
- Why do you take the medicine? What is its purpose?
- How often do you take it?
- Do you have a routine for taking it?
- Have you had any side effects from the medicine?
- Do you have any allergies to medicines?
- Do you buy or do you take any medicines which are not prescribed but have been bought from the chemist, shops or supermarket?
- Has anyone, a friend, neighbour or family member, lent or suggested you should take some of their prescribed medicines, homely remedies or vitamin or herbal products?
- Do you take any other forms of medication?

---

1 Barat, I., Andreason, F., Damsgaard, E. M. (2001). Drug therapy in the elderly: what doctors believe and patients actually do. *British Journal of Clinical Pharmacology*, **51**(6) 615–22.
2 Cantrill J. A, Sibbald, C., Buetow., S, (1998). Indicators of the appropriateness of long term prescribing in general practice in the United Kingdom: consensus development, face and content validity, feasibility and reliability. *Quality in Health Care*, **7**, 130–5.

Possible action following a review

- Patients/carers may need access to a prescriber or pharmacist to clear up any misconceptions.
- Provision of support items i.e. reminder charts, multi compartment aids, modified containers, large print labels.[3]
- Examine current diagnosis/ order investigations or additional monitoring and rationalise treatment according to clinical condition.

Box 8.1. Milestones for medicines management for older people[4]

Date	Action
2002	All people over 75 years should normally have their medication reviewed at least once a year and for those taking 4 or more medicines (polypharmacy) every 6 months.
	All hospitals to have a one stop dispensing/ dispensing for discharge scheme and, where appropriate, self administration schemes for older people.
2004	Every PCT will have schemes in place to enable older people to get more help from their pharmacists.

---

3 Raynor, D.K., Nicolson, M., Nunney, J., et al. (2000). The development and evaluation of an extended adherence support programme by community pharmacists for elderly patients at home. *International Journal of Pharmacy*, **8**, 157–64.
4 From: Department of Health (2001). *National Service Framework for Older people.* DOH, London.

Reflective practice

Why reflect?

Reflection in action and on action is now recognized as an essential tool to support safe and effective care delivery for all aspects of nursing.[1] Reflective practice is essential in supporting the analytical rationale for safe, effective, and appropriate prescribing.[2] Reflection links prescribing to continual professional development and to lifelong learning.

Reflection can be considered as a process critical to improving patient care and the process of critical reflection can be used to move practice forward. Written reflections can form part of a portfolio of prescribing practice which the prescriber may be called upon to provide to the NMC as evidence of continuing professional development and of safe and up-to-date practice. Reflection on prescribing should be considered an essential part of structured clinical supervision.

Models of reflection

There are several different models for reflection.[3] Choice of model of reflection depends on the individual prescriber's experience. The key models are listed below. It is essential that the reflector chooses a model which will best suit both their individual style and the subject matter on which they are reflecting. Some reflectors choose not to apply a model but prefer to reflect 'freestyle'.

Examples

The What? model of structured reflection (Driscoll)[4]
Kolb's model[5]
The Gibbs Reflective Cycle (Gibbs)[6]
- Description (What happened)?
- Feelings (What was I thinking and feeling)?
- Evaluation (What was good about the experience)?
- Analysis (What sense can I make of the experience)?
- Conclusion (What else could I have done)?
- Action plan (What would I do if it happened again)?

Reflecting on individual prescribing practice

PACT data (prescribing, analysis and cost[7] as issued by the Prescription Pricing Authority (PPA) can be useful for reflecting on group and individual prescribing practice. Reflective analysis of prescribing practice can be brought to clinical supervision and key reflective questions can be applied.

📖 Audit.
📖 Prescription analysis and cost (PACT).

1 Schon, C. (1987). Educating the Reflective Practitioners: How Professionals Think in Action. Temple Smith, London.
2 National Prescribing Centre (1999). Signposts for prescribing nurses – general principles of good prescribing. Prescribing Nurse Bulletin, Vol 1, N 10.
3 Atkins, S., Murphy, K. (1993). Reflection: a review of the literature. Journal of Advanced Nursing, **18**, 1188–92.
4 Driscoll, J. (2000) Practicing Clinical Supervision: a reflective approach. Ballière Tindall, London.
5 Kolb, D. (1984). Experiential Learning: experience as a source of learning and development. Prentice Hall, New Jersey.

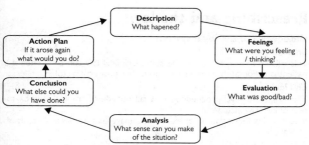

Adapted from Gibbs[6].

Questions to ask when reflecting on a prescribing incident:

- What (describe what happened)?
- How (describe the setting)?
- Why (what led up to the incident)?
- Why (why was the incident important)?
- What did you think at the time?
- What did you think after the incident?
- How did you feel during and after the incident?
- What was good about the incident?
- What was bad about the incident?
- How could the incident have occurred differently?
- What knowledge and skills did you use during the incident?
- What else could you have done?
- What more did you need to know?
- How could you have found the answers?
- What could you have done differently at the time?
- What would you do differently next time?
- Was anybody harmed or treated badly as a result of this incident?
- Having reflected on the above, what action do you now need to take?
- How will your reflection affect your actions next time?
- Do you have recommendations for future changes to practice?

6 Gibbs, G. (1988). Learning by doing. A guide to teaching and learning methods. Oxford Polytechnic Oxford.
7 British Medical Association and Royal Pharmaceutical Society of Great Britain. The British National Formulary (latest edn.) BMA, London.

Prescribing and the law

Categories of the legal system

Criminal law

This relates to crimes against the state. Criminal law can be broken if a patient is deliberately harmed, or if his or her property is stolen.

Civil law

This relates to legal proceedings that fall outside of criminal law. Examples of civil law include:

- tort (delict in Scotland): for example, damage that occurs as a result of negligence
- breach of contract.

Negligence

Practical examples of negligence:

- giving the wrong drug to the wrong patient
- giving the wrong drug to the right patient
- not doing something for a patient to alleviate suffering.

To avoid negligence when prescribing:

- check the drug
- check the patient
- question orders
- follow principles of prescribing
- seek supervision.

To succeed in a claim for negligence

The patient must demonstrate that:

- the nurse owed them a duty of care
- there was a breach in the duty of care
- harm occurred as a result of that breach.

The standard of proof is on the 'balance of probabilities' rather than 'beyond reasonable doubt'.

Vicarious liability

An employer is vicariously liable for his employee's negligent acts or omissions in the course of employment, whether authorized or not, unless the employer can show that the employee was undertaking 'a frolic of his own'[1] rather than the employer's business. The individual nurse still carries responsibility and, as such, is accountable for his or her actions.[2]

Competent standard of care

According to the Bolam principle (1957): the nurse is required to act within her or his competency at all times and to exercise 'the ordinary skill of an ordinary "man" exercising that particular art', i.e. perform reasonably as practitioners trained to the same standard within the same/similar professions, within a recognized standard of competency.[3]

1 per Park B in Joel v. Morrison, 1834, 6 C.&P. 501
2 NMC (2004). The NMC Code of Professional Conduct: Standards for Conduct, Performance and Ethics. NMC, London.
3 The quotation is from Bolam v Friern HMC, [1957] 1 WLR 582. Quoted in: Dimond, B. (2002). Legal aspects of nursing. (3rd edn). Prentice Hall, London.

Consent prescribing and the implications of parental responsibility

Consent for treatment can be given for a child by a person with parental responsibility for that child.

Definition

Parental responsibility covers all the rights, duties, and powers a parent has over a child and includes the right to consent to treatment.

Rights include the right to consent to treatment up until the child's eighteenth birthday.

Parental responsibility may be conferred automatically, i.e. a mother has this right conferred by law (Children Act 1989) on the birth of her child.

Or it may acquired by operation of the law, e.g a person who is appointed as the child's guardian or a local authority by obtaining a care order (Children Act 1989).

Children under 16

Children under the age of 16 years can give consent if it can be proven that they have a competent level of understanding. In Scotland, this is laid down in statute law[4] In England and Wales, it is expressed in the Fraser ruling.[5]

The age of consent for medical treatment in England and Wales is 16.[6]

📖 Legal differences between prescribing, administering, and dispensing.
📖 Safe prescribing.
📖 Prescribing for children.

Consent

To be valid, consent must be informed consent. Treating a patient without consent may constitute an assault and subject the nurse to damages for trespass to the person.

In the case of children, the court can overrule the wishes of the parent.[7]

---

4 Her Majesty's Stationary Office (1989). The Children Act. HMSO, London.
5 Age of Legal capacity (Scotland) Act 1991, section 2(4). See www.opsi.gov.uk/ACTS/acts1991
6 per Fraser LJ in Gillick v West Norfolk and Wisbech Area Health Authority and another, [1985] 3 All ER 402 at 413.
7 Family Law Reform Act 1969, section 8(1).

Ethics

Health care ethics are rooted in moral philosophy which tries to formulate sound arguments justifing our decisions and practices.

What is philosophy?

> [Philosophy] is something... is something intermediate between theology and science. Like theology it consists of speculation on matters, as to which definite knowledge has so far been unascertainable, but like science it appeals to human reason, rather than to (for example) divine authority... Between theology and science is a No Mans Land ... this No Mans Land is Philosophy.[1]

Some of the vocabulary of philosophy

Epistemology

The concept of what constitutes knowledge.

Asking questions such as:

- How can we differentiate knowledge from belief?
- Can sense or reason or intuition provide knowledge?
- Can we distinguish different types of knowledge e.g. practical, theoretical, moral aesthetic etc?

Ontology

Considers questions such as:

- Does the world exist independent of human thought?
- Is existence inseparable from thought?
- What is it to be a person?
- Does a person have free will?
- What is the nature of time?

Moral reasoning

Justifies decisions and practice on grounds of:

- **deontology** — justification on grounds of a moral duty to do good. (Deon is Greek for duty.)
- maintain the concept of obligation or a right to something are independent from the concept of good (i.e. some actions are right because they are intrinsically right).
- Immanuel Kant (1734–1804) was a proponent of deontology.
- the notions of beneficence and nonmaleficence are deontological theories (see NMC code of conduct).
- **consequentialism** — judgement is based on the amount of good generated by an action.
- **utilitarianism** is the most prominent Consequentialist theory.
- utilitarianism, founded by Hume, Bentham, and Mill in the 18th century maintains that the moral rightness of an action is determined by its good consequences, where goods might be the amount of pleasure, health, friendship, or knowledge the action generates (see Box 8.2).

---

1 Russell, B. (1946). History of Western Philosophy. Allen and Unwin, London.

Box 8.2 Examples of theoretical deontological and consequentialist decisions

(Remember our practice is governed by both ethical and legal decisions.)

Moral problem	Deontological argument (judged on duty)	Consequentialist argument (judged on outcome)
Telling the truth	Have a duty to always tell the truth regardless of the outcome. Therefore morally right to tell the truth.	It depends on the outcome of truth telling, it may cause harm and if it does it would be morally wrong.
Euthanasia	Life is sacred and therefore it is morally wrong to take it.	If it stops pain and suffering it would be a morally right act.
Informed consent	This is morally right as it respects autonomy.	It could be morally wrong, as it might frighten the patient and stop them having a life saving procedure.
Abortion	Life is sacred and to take it is morally wrong.	If it prevents suffering it is morally right.

Four principles which supply a framework for biomedical ethics

Autonomy — from the Greek *autos* (self) and *nomos* (rule or govern), it now encompasses such meanings as: self-governance, liberty, rights, privacy, and individual choice. Respect for autonomy is regarded as a duty and therefore is justified under the theory of Deontology.

An autonomous act has to have intentionality. It has to be done with understanding of the issues. and without influences that control or determine the action (see 12 key points on consent: the law in England).[1]

Nonmaleficence — it is morally wrong to inflict evil or harm.
Harm can be an injury that is physical, emotional, or financial.

Beneficence — the capacity of promoting and achieving good.
It may be applied to individuals or to society as a whole.

Justice — this encompasses notions of fairness and equity. It requires a system of universal rules and principles to ensure verifiable and transparent decisions are made. It also includes concepts of respect for autonomy, objectivity, and impartiality.

Four additional independent principles

These are justified on the basis of the preceding four principles.
- Promise keeping.
- Truthfulness
- Privacy
- Confidentiality

Consent

There are two distinct meanings of consent within the field of healthcare.
1. An autonomous action by the patient that authorizes the professional to involve the patient in research or to initiate a medical plan or intervention.
2. Within the term of social rules of consent it is used within institutions where it is legally necessary to obtain valid consent before proceeding with any therapeutic procedures or research.

Elements of informed consent:
- Full disclosure.
- Understanding — the individual patient's needs, knowledge of the purpose, and nature of the intervention, any likely effects or risks and the likelihood of success and any alternatives.
- Voluntariness.
- Competence.
- Consent.

---

1 Department of Health (2001). 12 key points on consent: the law in England. DoH, London.

NB. You can treat without consent in an emergency where the patient is unconscious and or the treatment cannot be safely delayed.

Box 8.3. Issues regarding consent

Issue	Advice
When the practitioner has the right to treat	<ul><li>Adults with a lack of capacity to decide for themselves.</li><li>Patients who are unable to consent or refuse medical treatment.</li><li>People with a long term mental disability or temporary lack of capacity.</li><li>Those who pass the best interest test.</li></ul>
Best interest test	<ul><li>Is it a case of necessity to save a life?</li><li>Will the action ensure an improvement in the patient's condition?</li><li>Will the action prevent a deterioration in the patient's condition?</li><li>In many cases it is not only lawful to treat but it is a doctor's duty to do so.</li><li>See NMC Code of Conduct[2]</li></ul>
Who can consent if the patient is unable to do so?	<ul><li>Relatives? — No (consult only to ascertain if there is a living will).</li><li>Doctor? — Yes if the best interest test is passed.</li><li>Court of law? — No.</li></ul>
A person's competency to consent	<ul><li>Need to be comprehending and retaining information.</li><li>Need to believe it.</li><li>Need to be able to weigh up the information.</li></ul>
Overriding refusal for consent.	<ul><li>Lack of capacity – non competence or undue influence.</li><li>Change in circumstances the time consent was given or withheld.</li></ul>

For more advice regarding consent see NMC Code of Conduct part 3, page 5[2].

2 Nursing and Midwifery Council. (2006) The NMC Code of Professional Conduct: Standards of Conduct, Performance and Ethics. NMC, London.

Rights

What is a right?
- An implied permission to follow a course of action.
- Restriction of what others may do.
- Creation of obligations to observe the right.

How do we enforce a right?
- Justified coercion
- Resistance
- Compensation
- Punishment.

What is a natural right?
- An obligation that is held by all (universal) e.g. the right to life.
- An obligation that is grounded in the nature of being a person, e.g. the right to respect of human dignity.

What is a negative right?
- The right to prohibit another from interference in your life, e.g. the right not to violated by theft or fraud.
- It can be respected by doing nothing at all.

Examples of a decision tree

What makes it morally wrong to kill?

It deprives another of their future.

Is there a time in early fetal development when it is acceptable to kill?

No, because it still deprives another of their future.

Therefore it is never morally justified to abort a fetus.

If we agree it is morally wrong to kill a person can we ask what is it to be a person?

We could argue that to be a person certain characteristics are needed:
–Consciousness
–Sentience
–Self F1 motivated activity etc.

It could be argued that a foetus does not have enough of these characteristics and therefore is not a person. So there is no moral imperative not to kill a foetus.

Accountability

According to the NMC, accountability is the professionally recognized term for responsibility for something or to someone.

Nurse prescribers are accountable for all aspects of:
- prescribing
- recommendation of an OTC product
- assessment
- decision making
- ensuring that the prescribed/recommended item is applied or administered as directed, either by the patient, their carers, the nurse, him/herself or any other person to whom the task is delegated.

Since accountability is an integral part of professional practice, the nurse prescriber has to be accountable, i.e. able to give an explanation of actions or omissions, to him/herself, the profession through the NMC, the patient, and to society as a whole.

Professional accountability

The NMC has set out guidelines for the administration of medicines and list the following requirements to be met for professional accountability. The prescriber must:
- Know the therapeutic use of the medication, the normal dosage. side effects, precautions, and contraindications.
- Be certain of the identity of the patient.
- Be aware of the patient's care plan.
- Have checked that the label and/or any directions supplied by the pharmacist are clear, correct, and unambiguous.
- Have considered the timing, dosage, and method of administration with regards to the patient's abilities and other co-existing therapies.
- Have checked the expiry date of the medicine to be administered.
- Have checked that the patient does not have any known allergies to the medication prior to administration.
- Ensure that if contraindications to a medicine are discovered, either when the patient has a reaction or when assessment indicates the unsuitability of the product, the prescriber or another authorized prescriber must be contacted without delay.
- Make clear, concise, and immediate signed and dated records of all medicines administered, intentionally withheld, or refused by the patient. The prescriber is responsible for record keeping even if the administration is delegated.
- Ensure that when supervising a student in medicine administration a clear countersignature must be given.

If a nurse fails to follow these guidelines, it is possible that the NMC will consider disciplinary action under its Code of Conduct.

When considering allegations of drug errors the NMC takes great care to discriminate between those cases where the error was the result of reckless or incompetent practice, or was concealed, and those that resulted from other causes such as serious pressure of work, and where there was an immediate honest disclosure in the patient's interest.[1]

1 Nursing and Midwifery Council (2002). Guidelines for the administration of medicines. NMC, London.

Indemnity

Indemnity is the legal term for protection. Nurse prescribers may be shielded from the consequences of a court case regarding actions or omissions if indemnity for those actions and omissions exist.

Liability

Liability is the legal term for responsibility and it is used to identify who was responsible for any harm which occurs as a result of clinical practice.

Criminal liability

- The Medicines Act 1968 describes exactly the permitted actions that can be taken by identified clinicians when prescribing.
- The Act also sets out penalties for any breaches of the strict wording of the legislation.
- Any such breach is a criminal offence.

Civil liability

- If a patient is harmed by a medication error, they may sue for negligence and ask a court to compensate them for the harm.
- The court will decide who is responsible by asking:
  - *Was there a duty of care?* Yes, if a nurse prescribes or administers a medication to a patient.
  - *Was the standard of care the same as a reasonable nurse would have provided?* An expert witness will be called to see if the standard of care was sufficient.
  - *Was the harm a direct result of the failure in delivery of a sufficient standard of care?* This is the most difficult part for the patient to prove as they must demonstrate that the injury was as a direct result of the failure in the standard of care and was not caused by the underlying condition being treated.

Protection for prescribers regarding accountability, responsibility, and liability

Vicarious liability

Vicarious liability may be explained as legal protection provided to employed staff working within agreed protocols or established and agreed methods by their employer, who is insured to cover claims.

The prescriber is protected from being sued for harming a patient because the law requires the employer to take legal responsibility for any acts or omissions on the part of the employee. The self-employed need to obtain personal insurance cover.

If you are working for a different practice perhaps as part of a flu immunization campaign, you need to check that you are still covered.

See also NMC Code of Conduct (2004) (section 9: Indemnity Insurance, pages 11 and 12).

Professional indemnity

- If a prescriber takes action outside agreed protocols or procedures, the employer may argue that vicarious liability does not apply.
- The prescriber will require professional indemnity insurance cover which will provide legal advice, representation, and, if appropriate, compensation.
- The main professional organizations (RCN, RMN, Unison, CDNA, and CPHVA) for example provide indemnity as part of their membership fee. (The RCN indemnifies current members for up to £3 million for each claim.)

Patient group directions (PGD)

History

Following questioning of the legality of group protocol practice,[1] a recommendation was made that protocols should offer practitioners the minimum of discretion and, in order to remain within the law, be patient specific. The government set out guidelines for the development of these protocols now to be called Patient Group directions (PGD).[2] The legal concerns were addressed by the Department of Health in a statutory instrument.[3]

Definition

Written instructions for the supply and administration of a named medicine to groups of individuals who may not be individually identified prior to presentation for treatment.

Further reading

Griffith, R. (2005). A nurse prescriber's guide to the legal implications of parental responsibility. *Nurse Prescribing*, **3** (3).

Nursing and Midwifery Council (2004). *Code of Professional Conduct.* Stationery Office, London

Nursing and Midwifery Council (2002). *Guidelines for the administration of medicines.* NMC, London.

Russell, B. (1939). *A History of Western Philosophy.* Allen & Unwin, London.

1 Department of Health (1998). Report on the Supply and Administration of Medicines under Group Protocols. (Crown part 1) Stationery Office, London.

2 Department of Health (2000). Patient Group directions (England Only) Health service Circular HSC2000/026, (9 August). DoH, Leeds.

3 Department of Health (2001). 12 key points on consent: the law and England. www.doh.gov.uk/consent, accessed 03.05.05.

Data Protection Act

Purpose

The purpose of the Data Protection Act 1998 is to ensure fair and lawful access to and processing of data. Personal data is both electronically and manually stored data which in the case of prescribing relates to the individual (patient or client).

There are eight principles which have been put into place by the act to ensure that information is handled properly.

Eight principles

The eight principles of the act state that data must be:
- fairly and lawfully processed
- processed for limited purposes
- adequate, relevant, and not excessive
- accurate
- not kept for longer than is necessary
- processed in line with your rights
- secure
- not transferred to countries without adequate protection.

The Act covers personal data which is held both in electronic format and manually if the data is held within a structured filling system which is relevant to the subject (patient/client).

> The Department of Health recommends that GP records are kept for a minimum of 10 years and recommends that hospital records are kept for a minimum of 8 years following the end of any treatment, or the patient's death if the patient died whilst receiving treatment. At the end of that specified time the health records would remain at the NHS Trust or in the case of GP health records, transferred to the relevant Primary Care Trust/Health Authority who will then make a decision as to whether to retain or destroy the records.[1]

If a patient moves abroad, they can make a request for their medical records under the Data Protection Act.

Those with proof of parental responsibility can request to access children's medical records. The legal age to give consent to medical treatment is sixteen however, if a child is deemed as having the capacity to make an informed decision, consent must first be obtained from that child before confidential information is shared.

📖 Record keeping.

---

1 Department of Health. (2006). Records Management: NHS Code of Practice. DoH, London.

Access to medical records

Patients have the right to obtain copies their medical records under the Data Protection Act 1998.[1] The records should be presented to the patient in a format that they will understand.

Legal exceptions to the right to access records exceptions include:

- where health professionals believe that the ability to access their records may seriously harm the patient or another person.
- information regarding other people – this may be removed from the records.
- access to records on behalf of a third party – this requires the subject's consent or power of attorney.

Records can be requested informally or formally. Formal application must be in writing and entitles applicants to a response within no more than forty days after the application has been made. The applicant will need to provide signed proof of identity. There is usually a charge ranging between £10–£50 when requesting access to records.

If access to medical records is refused, the applicant can appeal through the Information Commissioner's office telephone number in England: 01625 545745. Complaints about the service can be made through the health service ombudsman via www.ombudsman.org.uk

Human Rights Act (1998)

The rights of the individual are protected under the 1998 Human Rights Act[2] and apply to access to information, confidentiality, and the protection of family and private life. Prescribers have a duty of care to ensure that any records which they maintain with regards to individual patients are confidential.[3] There is the rare occasion when the prescriber may be called upon by the courts to disclose information which may be strongly in the interest of the public or which may support the proceedings of the prescriber's regulatory body or with the patient's specific consent for teaching or research purposes.

📖 Prescribing and the law.

Further reading

BBC Action Network (2005). How to access your medical records: http://www.bbc.co.uk/dna/actionnetwork/A1181657.

Department of Health (2003). Guidance for Access to Health Records Requests under the Data Protection Act 1998.

Mullan K. (2003). Supplementary Prescribing and Access to Medical Records: (2) Access Rights of Patients and Others. The Pharmaceutical Journal (Vol 271).

---

1 Her Majesty's Stationary Office (1998). *The Data Protection Act*. HMSO, London.
2 Her Majesty's Stationary Office (1998). *The Human Rights Act*. HMSO, London.
3 The Nursing and Midwifery Council (2004). *Code of Conduct and Ethics*. NMC, London.

Understanding research papers

Questions to ask when considering the evidence
- How many in subjects are in the trial?
- What are you measuring?
- What measurement tools are being used?
- Is the study a quantitative study?
- Is it a qualitative study?
- Is it a combination of both?
- How is data analysed?

Why do we need evidence?
- Governance and quality assurance
- Complex treatment regimens
- Geographical variation
- Established versus effective
- Expert patients
- Critical appraisal
- Resource allocation

📖 Evidence-based practice.

Weighing up the evidence/ points to consider
- Who told me about it?
- Cost versus risk benefit?

Questions to ask when evaluating the evidence
- What was the research question?
- Who sponsored the trial?
- Was the trial **randomized** and or **double blind**?
- How does the drug in question/intervention compare with other agents/interventions?
- How many participants were there?
- Was the trial population reflective of future potential user population?
- Methodology- Is the methodology clear and logical?
- Did the results produce **relevant outcome measurements**?
- Did the researchers produce **correct interpretation of results**?
- If it was a drug trial was there **an intention to treat analysis?**
- Were the conclusions **valid conclusions** in that they that reflected the results?
- Was the trial outcome relevant to the age group in the trial?
- How many participants were there in trials before the product was marketed?
- Are there reports of post marketing surveillance?

Desirable attributes for research trials
- Valid
- Cost-effective
- Reproducible
- Reliable
- Represents best interests of patient and professionals

- Clinically applicable
- Clinically flexible
- Clear
- Well documented
- Clear schedule for review
- Recommendations are made for sensible audit and or monitoring.

Best evidence

Gold Standard — randomized control trials (RCT)

Typology of supporting Evidence for Evidence Based practice (EBP) as used by National Service Frameworks (NSFs)

- A1: systematic reviews which contain at least one RCT e.g. systematic reviews from the Cochrane or Centre for Reviews and Dissemination.
- A2: other systematic and high quality reviews which synthesises references e.g. meta-analysis.
- B1: individualized RCTs.
- B2: individual non-randomized, experimental/interventional studies.
- B3: individual well-designed non-experimental studies, controlled statistically, if appropriate, includes studies using case control, longitudinal, cohort, matched pairs, or cross-sectional random sample methodologies and well-designed qualitative studies; well-designed analytical studies including secondary analysis.
- C1: descriptive and other research or evaluation not in B.
- C2: case studies and examples of good practice.
- D: summary review articles and discussions of relevant literature and conference proceedings not otherwise classified.

Evidence from expert opinion

- P: professional opinion based on clinical evidence, or reports of committees.
- U: user opinion.
- C: carer opinion.

Clinical trials

- In **Phase I trials**, researchers test a experimental drug or treatment in a small group of people (20–80) for the first time to evaluate its safety, determine a safe dosage range, and identify side effects.
- In **Phase II trials**, the experimental study drug or treatment is given to a larger group of people (100–300) to see if it is effective and to further evaluate its safety.
- In **Phase III trials**, the experimental study drug or treatment is given to large groups of people (1,000–3000) to confirm its effectiveness, monitor side effects, compare it to commonly used treatments, and collect information that will allow the experimental drug or treatment to be used safely.
- In **Phase IV trials**, post marketing studies delineate additional information including the drug's risks, benefits, and optimal use.

Some evidence-based guidelines
- **NICE** (National Institute for Clinical Excellence and Health)
- **SIGN** (Scottish Intercollegiate Guidelines Network)
- **BHS** (British Hypertension Society)
- **BDS** (British Diabetes Society).

Why use guidelines?
- Avoids prescribing from habit
- Guides new staff
- Improves patient confidence
- United front
- Time saving
- Governance
- Standardized practice
- New therapies
- Educational tools
- Familiarity.

Points to consider when implementing guidelines
- Workload and practice implications?
- Resources?
- The need to improve skill?
- Implications for patient?
- Computer support?
- Dissemination?

Table 8.1 Explanation of research design terms

Research term	Explanation	Some flaws found in study designs
RCT	Study design where treatment, interventions, or enrolment into different study groups are assigned by random allocation. If the sample size is large enough, this design avoids bias and confounding variables.	No power calculation for group sizes lower than 20. No blinding of outcome measurement.
Systematic review	An approach based on a strategy, which has clear inclusion and exclusion criteria. Aims to detect biases, random errors, unsupported claims in the methodology, interpretation of results, and content.	No explicit assessment of validity of included study. Studies combined inappropriately.
Descriptive study	Describes the distribution of variables within a group.	Can be subjective.
Experimental studies	Allocation or assignment is under the control of the investigator.	Unblinded.
Intervention studies	Observation of the effect of an intervention.	Unblinded.
Case study	Focuses on the situation, dynamics and complexity of a single case or compares a small number of cases.	Inclusion/exclusion criteria need to be stated, justified and adhered to.
Qualitative study	Research which is carried out in the real world and is analysed in non-statistical ways.	Analysis and interpretation procedures are often unclear. Interpretations not explicitly based on data.

Further Reading

Bero, L., Grilli, R., Grimshaw, J.M., et al. (1998). Getting research findings into practice: closing the gap between research and practice: an overview of systematic reviews of interventions to promote the implementation of research findings. BMJ, **317**: 465–468.

Crombie, I. K. (1996). The pocket guide to critical appraisal. BMJ books, London.

Greenhalgh, T. (1997). Assessing the methodological qualities of published papers. BMJ, **315**, 305–8.

Grol R, Dalhuijsen J et al. (1998). Attributes of clinical guidelines that influence the use of guidelines in general practice. BMJ, **317**: 858–861.

Walsh K, Ham C, (1997). Acting on the evidence: progress in the NHS. NHS Confederation.

▣ www.jr2.ox.ac.uk/bandolier.

Part III

Practice

Working as a nurse prescriber

Working as a nurse prescriber

Accountability
- You are accountable for prescribing acts and omissions.
- You are personally accountable for each prescription you write.
- Keep up to date with competencies.
- Work only within your competencies and within the remit of your job description.
- Only prescribe if you have seen the patient.
- Resist the pressure from others to prescribe.
- Seek regular clinical supervision.

Questions to answer prior to and on qualifying
- Have you identified a Trust prescribing lead?
- Is there a Trust policy or guidelines for prescribing?
- Will you be covered by your employers under vicarious liability? (Remember that you may also be personally liable.)
- Is a mechanism for continual professional development in place?
- Are your prescribing needs addressed through the HR review mechanism?
- How are you going to keep up to date?
- Are you a member of a professional body that supports/informs your prescribing?
- How are you going to prove that you are keeping your competencies sharp?
- Are there other prescribers with whom you can seek supervision/ network?
- Have you informed your medical colleagues of your ability to prescribe?
- Have you negotiated a mechanism and local working agreement to prescribe?
- Do you have appropriate professional liability insurance (PLI)?
- Does your PLI cover prescribing?

On qualifying
- Notify the Trust prescribing lead of your qualification.
- Ensure that prescription pads are ordered.
- Provide the Trust lead with a specimen of your signature.
- Provide local pharmacies with specimens of your signature (primary care).
- Provide hospital pharmacies with specimens of your signature (secondary care).

Prescribing from the BNF
- Prescribe within the limitations of your competency.
- You cannot prescribe unlicensed drugs as a nurse independent prescriber.
- You can prescribe a limited range of controlled drugs as a V300 independent nurse prescriber. These are listed in the drug tariff.
- Keep up-to-date with changes to the formulary.

- Keep up-to-date with developments in prescribing practice.
- Keep up-to-date with changes to prescribers' remit.
- Prescribe according to local formulary and local policy.

It is a good practice to maintain your portfolio of prescribing practice.

Questions to ask before prescribing

- Have you informed your colleagues of your new role?
- Have you informed your patients/clients of your new role?
- How have you informed the above?
- How has this information been received?
- Is the software in place to support your prescribing?
- Do your employers have electronic systems that 'talk to each other'?
- Are there recognized templates for CMPs?
- Are templates for CMPs adaptable to the needs of individual patients?
- Do you have prescription pads with your identifier on them (primary care)?
- Do you have drug charts that have been amended to include the signature of the nurse prescriber?
- Does the pharmacy have a sample of your signature?
- Do you have access to shared electronic records?
- Does your patient have patient-held records?
- Do you have Internet access?
- Do you have access to key prescribing web sites?

Questions I need to ask myself before prescribing

These pages have been left blank for the reader to complete

Prescribing legally from the British National Formulary

Legal classification of medicines: the classification can relate to the pack size that is being sold.
- **Prescription only medicines (POMs)**: can only be supplied and dispensed if a prescription is issued by a legally qualified prescriber or under a patient group direction,[1] e.g. 100 paracetamol.
- **Pharmacy only/over the counter (P) medicines**: products that are for sale as supervised by a registered pharmacist e.g. 32 paracetamol.
- **General sales list products**: available from shops other than pharmacies, such as petrol stations and supermarkets, e.g. 16 paracetamol.
- **Over the counter medicines** (OTC) are a colloquial term for medicines which can be purchased without the need for a prescription or on advice from a pharmacist.

Prescribing legally from the BNF
- Prescribe only within your competency area.
- The drugs and appliances must be listed within the BNF.
- Write prescriptions only for the route or form as indicated by the BNF.

---

1 British Medical Association and Royal Pharmaceutical Society of Great Britain. *British National Formulary* (latest edn). BMA, London.

Physical exams and history taking

History taking

A thorough history and physical examination are fundamental before prescribing for any patient. The purpose of history taking is to gather information from the patient to establish a trusting and supportive relationship with them in order to provide holistic care.

📖 Holistic assessment.

You will need to record:
- The date and time.
- Identifying data for the patient: age, gender, marital status, and occupation.
- Source of history or referral:
- Information from the patient, friend, family carer, etc.
- Reliability of information if relevant
- Chief complaints—where possible in the patient's own words
- Present illness, including:
  - Location of the complaint—where is it?
  - Does it move?
  - Quality—what is it like?
  - Quantity or severity—how bad is it?
  - Timing—when does it start?
  - How long does it last?
  - How often does it occur?
  - Setting – environmental factors:
    –which activities are associated with the complaint?
    –are there any emotional reactions which may have contributed to this illness?
    –are there factors that make it worse or better?
  - Other associated manifestations
- Current medications including homely remedies, over the counter medications (OTC), herbs, or medicines products borrowed from another person (📖 OTC medications).
- Any known allergies.
- Identify any red flag symptoms.
- Past history:
  - childhood illnesses
  - adult illnesses
- Current health status:
  - smoker?
  - alcohol, drugs, and or related substance abuse?
  - other risk taking leisure activities
  - exercise and diet
  - immunizations
  - screening tests
- Family history:
  - note the age and health or age and death of each immediate family member. Information regarding the health of grandparents or grandchildren may also be of use.

- note the occurrence within the family of any disease.
    e.g. diabetes, stroke, heart disease.
- Personal and social history:
    - occupation and education
    - home situation and significant others
    - daily life
    - important experiences
    - religious/spiritual beliefs.

📖 Using models of consultation for prescribing.
📖 Clinical and physical examination.

Clinical or physical examination

A structured and systematic approach needs to be taken to make a diagnosis, as outlined by the National Prescribing Centre (NPC): '[the nurse prescriber] takes a comprehensive medical history and undertakes the appropriate physical examination'.[1]

Information needs to be gathered from three main sources:
- history taking
- physical/clinical examination
- appropriate investigations.
📖 History taking

In addition to the comprehensive verbal history which will be taken by the practitioner, prompting the patient to describe their experience of the presenting condition in a clear and factual way, close observation of the patient's physical and clinical condition is required.

Note and record, as part of the assessment, the patient's:
- appearance
- movement
- demeanour.

Remember, a patient may be concerned about their tiredness and not think of swelling in their ankles and breathlessness as important. You will need to note these symptoms and address them after taking the patient's history.

Most provisional diagnoses will be made by the end of the history-taking process.

Clinical examination
- Further evidence in order to support or reject the provisional diagnosis will be gained by examining the patient.
- The physical areas examined will depend on the provisional diagnosis.
- It is important, however, to return to the history taking if the findings on examination do not support the provisional diagnosis.
- Always be sensitive to the patient's:
  - dignity
  - concerns
  - religious and cultural needs.

Remember
- You are legally required to ask the patient's permission to carry out a physical examination.
- Do not do anything outside your area of competence; always consider your training and experience.

Further reading
Bates, B., Bickley, I.S., Hoekelman, M.D. (1996). *Physical examination and history taking* (6th edn). J.B. Lippincott, Philadelphia.

1 National Prescribing Centre (2003). 🖥 www.npc.co.uk

Using models of consultation for prescribing

Consulting for prescribing

Models of consultation have been developed to support practice. A model can be viewed as a structural framework around which to build effective practice. To prescribe safely, you must develop and practise a safe, holistic, and effective consultation style. Patient/practitioner consultations have traditionally been medically led and, as such, paternalistic—the professional is in control of the consultation to which the patient is a passive recipient

Patients' choices within the consultation are affected by their 'health beliefs'. Health beliefs are influenced by many variables which must be viewed within the patient's cultural context. The health beliefs model[1] reviewed these as:

- the influence of the patient's social class, ethnicity, and personality
- the patient's perception of the severity of the disease threat
- the patient's perception of the risk/benefit of seeking treatment
- catalysts for action, e.g. severity of symptoms, pressure from family, information in the media.

Practitioner- and patient-centred models (adapted from Neighbour[2])

Using the disease–illness model,[3] the patient's condition is viewed as their primary concern and it is the task of the practitioner to assist the patient in seeking a remedy. Information is gathered from the perspective of both the patient and the practitioner, integration of both agendas leads to shared decision making and understanding.

Stott and Davis[4] suggested a systematic style of consultation which explored:

- management of presenting problems
- modification of help-seeking behaviours, e.g. educating the patient in self-help methods
- management of continuing problems, e.g. looking at long-term problems and solutions
- opportunistic health promotion, e.g. screening, vaccination, brief intervention for smoking cessation.

1 Becker, M.H., Maiman, L.A. (1975). Sociobehavioural determinants of compliance with medical care recommendations. *Medical Care*, **13**, 10–24.
2 Neighbour, R. (1997). *The inner consultation*. Petrock Press, Reading.
3 Stewart, M., Roter, D. (ed.) (1989). *Communicating with medical patients*. Sage Publications, Newbury Park, California.
4 Stott, N., Davis, R.H. (1979). The exceptional potential in each primary care consultation. *Journal of the Royal College of General Practitioners*, **29**, 201–5.

Pendleton et al.[5] detailed seven tasks that would lead to a structured and effective consultation:
1. Find out why the patient has come.
2. Are there any other problems?
3. In mutual doctor–patient consultation, act to address the problems.
4. Work to achieve a mutual understanding of the problems.
5. Involve the patient and encourage responsibility taking.
6. Efficient use of time and resources.
7. Establish and maintain an ongoing relationship with the patient.

Byrne and Long[6] described six phases that provided a logical framework for a consultation (adapted from Neighbour[2]):
Phase 1: Establishing a relationship.
Phase 2: Attempting to discover, or discovering, why the patient is consulting.
Phase 3: Conducting a verbal or physical examination.
Phase 4: Mutual consideration of the condition.
Phase 5: Practitioner-led or joint detailing of the need for further treatment or investigation.
Phase 6: Practitioner-led termination of the consultation.

Heron[7] categorized the interventions of practitioners into six main styles:
1. *Prescriptive*: using a directive, advice-giving approach.
2. *Informative*: sharing new knowledge, explaining this to the patient.
3. *Confronting*: challenging existing attitudes and beliefs within a supportive environment.
4. *Cathartic*: supporting the patient to release emotions.
5. *Catalytic*: supporting patient exploration of thoughts and feelings.
6. *Supportive*: comforting the patient and affirming their value.

Heron's model can be argued to be consumerist, in that the patient makes demands of the practitioner which are based on actual and perceived need. The patient is in control of the consultation.

Neighbour[2] categorized patient–practitioner consultation into five useful checkpoints:
1. *Connecting*: establishing a practitioner–patient rapport.
2. *Summarizing*: listening to the patient, eliciting information.
3. *Handover*: mutual agreement/decision making and action.
4. *Safety netting*: checking that all key points have been covered, setting in place processes for record keeping, review, and reflection.
5. *Housekeeping*: caring for the needs of the practitioner.

In this model there is a mutuality/partnership – both parties have shared and equal control. This style is based on shared respect and works well for situations when negotiating a contract.

📖 Holistic assessment.
📖 History taking.

5 Pendleton et al. (1984). The consultation: an approach to learning and teaching. Oxford University Press, Oxford.
6 Byrn. P., Long. B. (1976). *Doctors Talking to Patients*. HMSO, London.
7 Heron, J. (1975). Six category intervention analysis. Human Potential Research Project, University of Surrey.

Communication

The purpose of effective patient-centred communication in relation to prescribing is to promote concordance. Patient-centred communication takes into account the patient's:
- hopes
- beliefs
- attitudes
- expectations.

📖 Concordance.

The patient's agenda may differ from that of the prescriber. To prescribe effectively, listening must be balanced with the gathering of information:
- the patient's perception of the problem may be different from that of the prescriber
- the patient may not be telling you the full story
- the problem that they present with may not be the problem they wish you to treat.

Effective communication: the role of the prescriber
- Respect the patient.
- Respect the patient's agenda.
- Be sensitive to the patient.
- Listening supportively.
- Show sensitive body language.
- Empathize.
- Establish the patient's hopes, fears, and expectations.
- Clarify.
- Listen actively.
- Ask open-ended questions.
- Give accurate feedback.
- Gather all of the information.
- Ask the patient to fill in the gaps.
- Analyse the information.
- Seek the truth (perceived and actual).
- Give factual and easily interpreted evidence-based information.
- Explain all options.
- Explain the effects of drug.
- Explain side effects.
- Negotiate efficiently.
- Communicate at a pace that is appropriate for your individual patient.

Communicating with the wider team
- Ensure that others who are caring for the patient are kept up to date with changes to the patient's prescriptions.
- Information can be communicated via patient-held records and by shared electronic records.

📖 Record keeping.

Equity and communication

Consider:

- effective communication for people for whom English is not their first language
- effective communication for those with audio or visual impairment
- effective communication for those with learning disabilities.

Web sites to support communication with patients who are audio or visually impaired and for those with learning disabilities:

Royal National Institute for the Blind 🖥 www. rnib.org.uk
Royal National Institute for the Deaf 🖥 www.rind.org.uk
🖥 www.doh.co.uk _ learning disabilities link
🖥 www.mencap.org.uk

Ensuring an effective consultation

Proceed in a sequence that is logical to yourself and to your patient.[1]

Before the consultation

- Ensure that there is adequate time set aside to prepare for the consultation.
- Read the patient's records.
- Anticipate the patient's agenda, but do not set it for them.
- Give yourself space between patients.
- Tidy your desk space.
- Prepare the necessary documents and necessary equipment.
- Anticipate how long you will need to be able to complete the consultation.

Remember that first impressions count

To develop a relationship you need to employ verbal and non-verbal communication and to involve the patient at each stage of decision making.

- Greet the patient.
- Ensure that you have got the right patient.
- Ask the patient to introduce themselves.
- Make eye contact.
- Make your patient comfortable.
- Establish a mutuality/rapport.
- Attend to their basic needs.
- Identify the purpose of the consultation.
- Explain and clarify your role.
- Introduce yourself by name and role.
- Clarify why the patient has come to see you.
- Explain what you do.
- Ask the patient what he expects from the consultation.
- Look for other underlying reasons for the patient to be attending the consultation.

Consider your patient

- Does your patient feel at ease?
- Are they comfortable?
- Why have they come?
- What do they want from the consultation?
- Can they talk to you?
- Is there mutual respect?
- Let the patient set the agenda.
- Is it the same as yours?
- Be aware of the patient's facial expressions and body language.
- Listen initially without interrupting.
- Use open questions to keep the consultation moving and closed ones to bring it to a controlled help

📖 History taking.

1 Kurtz, S.M., Silverman, J.D., Draper, J. (1998). Teaching and learning communication skills. Radcliffe Medical Press, Oxford.

Record keeping

Follow the NMC's Standards for record keeping.[1]
- Record prescribing decisions in patient-held records (if available) and in shared medical notes (paper or electronic) as in standard practice.
- Ensure contemporaneous record keeping with a maximum time lapse of 24–48 hrs and 72 hrs on bank holidays.

📖 Data protection.

What to record
- The time, date, and purpose of the consultation.
- Outcome of negotiated decision-making.
- If you have prescribed or recommended medication to be bought from the pharmacist or as general sales list medication.
- Instructions you have given the patient.
- Dose, frequency, how often, and how long to take medication for.
- What you have advised the patient to do in the event of unexpected side effects.
- Date of proposed review.

Negotiation within the team
Inform fellow professionals of your role as a nurse prescriber.

It is important to maintain patient confidentiality but, in the interest of safe prescribing, other prescribers and clinicians who have access to the patient's medical records must be informed of prescribing decisions.
- In the case of supplementary prescribing, other prescribers can have access to a shared clinical management plan and, through access for professionals, to shared electronic records (where they are available).
- Patients and carers must be involved in negotiated decision-making and information should be recorded in patient-held records where available.
- Prescribing decisions must be documented in nursing notes, along with a copy of the clinical management plan.
- Avoid duplicating information that is already in the patient's notes.
- It is good practice to give a patient/carer a copy of the agreed clinical management plan.

Out of hours
It is vital that professionals who are involved in out-of-hours care have as near to contemporaneous as is possible access to medical records which must clearly document prescribing decisions.

📖 NMC code.

---

1 Nursing and Midwifery Council (2001). *Guidelines for records and record keeping.* NMC, London.

Using the British National Formulary (BNF)

The BNF is revised, updated, and published on a six-monthly basis and informs the prescriber about 'the selection, prescribing, dispensing and administration of medicines'.[1] Information is linked to clinical conditions. The BNF, along with other commercially produced formularies and locally produced NHS formularies, contains information regarding dosages, formulations, and pack sizes, as well as the market cost of the drug/appliance.

Guidance provided by BNF

- Prescription writing.
- Prescribing controlled drugs.
- Prescribing for dependencies.

Each edition of the BNF indicates any significant changes that have been made since the previous edition, including:
- dose changes
- classification changes
- discontinued preparations
- new preparations
- name changes of drugs to conform to European law.

The inside cover of the BNF contains useful contact numbers.
- Regional and District Medicines Information Services
- United Kingdom Medicines Information Pharmacists Group (UKMIPG)
- Driver and Vehicle Licensing Agency (DVLA)
- UK sport
- Poisons information services
- Travel information contact numbers.

The main text of the BNF is divided into 15 chapters to cover comprehensive prescribing for each system of the body and related clinical conditions.

Non-medical prescribers' formularies within the BNF include:
- nurse prescribers' formulary for community practitioners (CPF)
- dental practitioners' formulary

Information regarding controlled drugs and the drug tarrif which can be prescribed by nurse independent prescribers can be found at www.doh.gov.uk/nurseprescribing

As well as general information on prescribing, the BNF provides information on:
- prescription writing
- emergency supply of medicines
- controlled drugs and drug dependence
- adverse reactions to drugs
- prescribing for children

---

1 British Medical Association and Royal Pharmaceutical Society of Great Britain. *British National Formulary*, (latest edn). BMA, London.

- prescribing in palliative care
- prescribing for the elderly
- drugs and sport
- emergency treatment of poisoning
- index of manufacturers, contact addresses, and telephone numbers
- Joint British Societies Coronary Risk Prediction Charts
- adult advanced life support.

Appendices at the back of the BNF cover:
- drug interactions
- liver disease
- renal impairment
- pregnancy
- breast-feeding
- intravenous additives
- borderline substances
- wound management products and elastic hosiery
- cautionary and advisory labels for dispensed medicines.

Cautionary labels

The pharmacist who supplies and dispenses the medication is required to supply it with the recommended informative wording and, if necessary, a cautionary label. Wording for cautionary labels can be found inside the back cover of the BNF.

Abbreviations and symbols

Wherever possible, the BNF uses internationally recognized abbreviations and symbols. A list of abbreviations, symbols, Latin abbreviations, and E numbers, which are present in some medications, can be found inside the back cover of the BNF.

Yellow card reporting (adverse drug reactions)

Detachable yellow cards for the reporting of adverse drug reactions (ADRs) to the Committee on Safety of Medicines (CSM) can be found at the back of the BNF. Yellow card reporting can also be filed on line via 🖫 www.mhra.gov.uk

Prescribing for special groups

Prescribing for older people

It is important to accept the diversity and individuality of the people who make up the group catagorized as older people. This term has been described as a mask which is economically and socially constructed and brings with it many disadvantages. However, for the purpose of this section we will take older people as those with a chronological age over 60 years.

- Four in five people over the age of 75 years take at least one prescribed medicine, with 36% taking four or more medicines.[1]
- Polypharmacy is defined as being prescribed four or more medicines[2] and brings an increased risk of drug interaction and/or adverse drug reaction (ADR).
- Between 6 and 17% of older patients experience an ADR during their stay in hospital[3] and ADRs are implicated in between 5 and 17% of hospital admissions for those aged over 65 years.[4]

Holistic assessment

It is important to assess not only the presenting problem but also the altered pharmacodynamics and kinetics, which are part of the ageing process, as well as any underlying pathologies and/or polypharmacy.

Always check the use of herbal remedies, 'homely remedies', and OTC medication for possible drug interactions and food–drug interactions:

  Holistic assessment.

Common food–drug interactions[3]

Food	Drug	Action
Orange juice (vitamin C)	Iron sulphate	Enhances the absorption of iron
Dairy produce	Tetracycline	Reduces the absorption of tetracycline
Foods rich in tyramine, e.g. cheese, meat extract, some alcohol	Monoamine oxidase inhibitors	Toxic effect such as sudden hypertensive crisis
Pineapple or grapefruit juice	Warfarin	Enhances the anticlotting activity

1 Department of Health (1998) *Health Survey for England*. vol 1: Findings. Stationary Office, London. Available at: www.doh.gov.uk/nsf/medicinesop
2 Department of Health (2001) *NSF for older people*. Stationary Office, London. Available at: www.doh.gov.uk/nsf
3 Additional information regarding food/drug interactions: http://vm.cfsan.fda.gov~lrd/fdinter.html
4 Courtney, M., Butler, M. (2002). *Essential Nurse Prescribing*. GMM, London.

- Nurse prescribers should have some knowledge of common food–drug interactions and the implications these have on the timing of drug use.[4]
- Home circumstances, such as bereavement and a fear of expense, may cause older people to delay seeking help.
- Older people often have atypical symptoms or are stoical, which may lead them to under-report pain or depression.

Some practical aspects of prescribing for older people

Problem	Result	Possibility
A frail older person may have difficulty in swallowing	Tablets remain in the mouth, causing: • localized ulceration	Consider prescribing as a liquid Encouraging sufficient fluid to facilitate swallowing
	• slowed availability of the drug	Ensure the correct fluid, e.g. take with milk or take with water
Problems removing medications from the packs	Prescribed items not taken	Blister packs may be problematic, consider: • foil-packed tablets • using a compartmenta-lized box with daily doses in each section
Difficulties reading the label	Missed doses or taken at inappropriate times Overdose ADR	Use large-print labels in black and white
Forgetting to take medication	Missed doses	Consider using: • a compartmentalized box with daily doses in each section • a medicine reminder chart
Sensitivity to commonly used drugs	Nervous system may be sensitive to: • opioid analgesics • benzodiazepines • antipsychotics • antiparkinsonian drugs	Use with caution

📖 Basic principles of pharamcology.

Problems in prescribing for older people

Altered pharmacodynamics

📖 Basic principles of pharamcology.

Problems regarding the metabolism and excretion of drugs.

- Delayed metabolism by the liver and excretion by the kidneys results in prolonged drug action:
  - excretion by the kidneys requires a blood flow of 1500ml/min and a glomerular filtration rate (GFR) of 100ml/min
  - older people may have a GFR below 50 ml/min which, because of reduced muscle mass, may not be indicated by a raised serum creatinine
  - it is recommended to assume at least mild renal impairment when prescribing (📖 p.46).
- Complicated regimens may cause confusion and lead to excessive doses or overdose.
- Patients who are malnourished will have altered drug metabolism and distribution:
  - reduced plasma protein may mean there is an increase in the amount of drug available for activity
  - insufficient dietary protein may lead to reduced enzyme activity and slow the metabolism of a drug
  - a leaner body mass, with reduced fat stores, limits the sequestration of a drug in the fatty layers, increasing the amount actively available.

Altered pharmacokinetics

Caused by a decline in:
- body mass
- body fat stores
- total body water—this decreases by 10–15% between 20 and 80 years of age
- renal mass
- hepatic blood flow—with age hepatic blood flow and mass decrease
- glomerular filtration—the number of nephrons decreases with age and they become less efficient.

Renal clearance is reduced as a natural process of ageing, resulting in drugs being excreted more slowly and an increase in the susceptibility to nephrotoxic preparations.

This reduction in renal clearance is exacerbated by fairly routine illnesses, such as renal track infection (RTI) or urinary track infection (UTI), leading to the development of adverse effects or overdose in a patient previously stabilized on a drug with a narrow therapeutic margin (e.g. digoxin).

First-pass metabolism may be reduced, resulting in increased bioavailability.

Improving prescribing for older people

The NSF sets out the following milestones to improve prescribing practice for this age group:

- since 2002: all people over 75 years should normally have had their medicines reviewed at least annually, and those taking more than four medicines should have a 6-monthly review .
- all hospitals should have 'one stop dispensing/dispensing for discharge' schemes and, where appropriate, self-administration schemes for medicines for older people.
- since 2004: every PCT should have schemes in place so that older people get more help from pharmacists in using their medicines.[1]

Further reading

Royal College of Physicians (2000). *Sentinel: Clinical audit of evidence based prescribing for older people.* RCP, London.

1 Department of Health (2001) *NSF for older people.* Stationary Office, London. ▦ Available at: www.doh.gov.uk/nsf

Prescribing for public health

Public Health is defined by Acheson[1] as 'the science and art of preventing disease, prolonging life and promoting health through the organized efforts of society'. There is a widening gap between the rich and the poor in society.

Social determinants of health

A person's ability to attain a standard of health and well-being is influenced by their genetic make up and their lifestyle choices such as:
• diet
• exercise
• sexual behaviour.

The wider determinants of health include:
• housing
• employment
• transport
• education
• environment
• income
• social class
• ethnic origin.

Biological determinants include environmental hazards and infectious diseases.

The Government white paper 'Saving Lives: Our Healthier Nation'[2] aims to set in place strategies which will prevent 300,000 premature deaths by 2010. 'Saving Lives' set national priorities to improve health in the key target areas of:
• cancer
• coronary heart disease and stroke
• accidents
• mental health.

Targets were to be met through the implementation of health improvement plans (HIMPs) at a local health service trust level and by the introduction of health action zones (HAZs) in areas at increased risk of higher levels of disease and accidents.

NICE has set national guidelines for evidence-based best practice and the Department of Health has implemented NSFs which have set long term strategies to improve health and healthcare. The achievement of these strategies is currently measured by targets and standards are audited against best practice locally and nationally.

---

1 Department of Health (1998a). *The Independent Inquiry into Inequalities in Health Report.* Chairman: Sir Donald Acheson. The Stationary Office, London.
2 Department of Health (1999a). *Saving Lives: Our Healthier Nation.* The Stationary Office, London.

It is the aim of the Department of Health, through the implementation of NSFs and through NICE, to significantly decrease mortality and morbidity and to provide equitable standards of healthcare nationally. The rolling programme of NSFs first implemented in 1998 currently covers:

- children
- renal conditions
- long-term conditions
- diabetes
- older people
- mental health
- paediatric intensive care
- cancer
- coronary heart disease.

The NHS plan[3] set the template for a health service providing high quality care which is designed around the patient.

Opportunities for nurse prescribing and public health

- Greater patient choice
- Patient empowerment
- Reduced waiting times
- Improvements in local hospitals and surgeries
- Introduction of national standards
- New ways of working[4]
- Chief nursing officers ten key roles[5]
- Breakdown of barriers which demark roles[6].

Vaccination as a means of disease prevention

The latest version of the BNF has an up-to-date list of vaccinations which can be prescribed to prevent disease. See also 'Immunisation against Infectious Disease'[7] which reflects the advice of the Joint Committee on Vaccination and Immunisation (JCV) and which can be obtained online at: www.doh.gov.uk/greenbook.

Prevention of chronic/long-term conditions

Smoking cessation advice has been proven to be an economical and effective intervention for the prevention of many long-term conditions[8].
📖 Substance misuse and dependency.

3 Department of Health (2000a). *The National Health Service Plan*. The Stationary Office, London.
4 Department of Health (1999b). Making a Difference: Strengthening the Nursing, Midwifery and Health Visiting Contribution to Health and Health Care. HMSO, London.
5 Department of Health (2002). *Liberating the Talents*. Department of Health, London.
6 Naidoo, J., Wills, J. (2000). *Health promotion: foundation for practice* (2nd edition). Baillière Tindall, London. 📖 www.prodigy.nhs.uk/guidance
7 Department of Health (1996). Immunization against infections disease. 📖 Available at: www.doh.gov.uk/greenbook.
8 Department of Health (2000b). *Smoking Kills: a white paper on tobacco*. The Stationary Office, London.

Over prescribing of antibiotics

There is considerable concern about the over prescribing of antibiotics for the treatment of simple and self-limiting conditions. The Standing Medical Advisory Committee (SMAC) Sub-group on Antimicrobial Resistance[9] sought to reduce antibiotic usages and to promote international cooperation and consensus on the prescribing of antimicrobial drugs. Antibiotic use has been demonstrated to:

- select for bacterial resistance which spreads from one bacteria to another
- lengthen the patient's stay in hospital due to increase in complications.

Hospital prescribing accounts for 20% of prescribing for antimicrobial agents.[9] As a result of the increase in bacterial resistance to antimicrobial drugs, antibiotics are becoming less effective in the treatment of bacterial infections. There is mounting concern about the increasing resistance to antimicrobial agents of organisms such as *Mycobacterium* tuberculosis, *Streptococcus* pneumonia and *Neisseria* gonorrhea. The over prescribing of antibiotics for such conditions has led to antimicrobial resistance and to an increased threat of adverse drug reactions. Hospital acquired infections such as strains of *Staphylococcus aureus* and *Pseudomonas aerigonosa* are resistant to all antimicrobial agents.[10] Resistance to antifungal and antiviral agents is also developing.

Responsibilities of the nurse prescriber when prescribing for infectious disease

- Resist pressure to prescribe antibiotics unnecessarily.
- Educate the public to change their expectations.

SMAC (1998) recommendations

- No prescribing of antibiotics for simple coughs and colds.
- No prescribing of antibiotics for viral sore throats.
- Limit prescribing for uncomplicated cystitis to 3 days in otherwise fit women.
- Limit prescribing of antibiotics over the telephone to exceptional cases.

Other factors which influence antimicrobial resistance

- Hygiene.
- Infection control and cross infection.
- Veterinary and agricultural use.
- Industrial use.

Further recommendations

- Adherence to and harmonization between national and local prescribing evidence-based guidelines.
- International cooperation.
- Surveillance of resistance.
- Research.
- Education.
- Hygiene, infection controls and limitation of cross infection.[10]

---

9 Standing medical advisory committee. Report of sub-group on antimicrobial resistance. The path of least resistance. Department of Health, London.
10 Department of Health (2003). Winning Ways: Working Together to Reduce Healthcare Associated Infection in England. HMSO, London.

📖 Prescribing and sexual health.
📖 Prescribng for infections.
📖 Substance misuse and dependency.
📖 Sexual health.
See latest version of BNF

Further reading

British Medical Association and Royal Pharmaceutical Society of Great Britain (latest edition) *British National Formulary* No 49. BMA, London.

Prescribing for children

Safety

Pharmacokinetics and pharmacodynamics are often different for children than for adults and this can have surprising effects on the absorption, distribution, and metabolism of certain drugs. Refer to the *BNF for Children* which provides advice on the prescribing, dispensing, monitoring and administration of medicines to children of all ages.[1]

    Basic principles of pharmacology.
    Seven principles of safe prescribing.

NB: always seek expert advice if unsure when prescribing for children. As in all prescribing, only prescribe within your field of competency.

Key points

- Be hypervigilant when prescribing for neonates (babies under 30 days old).
- Allow for developmental differences in children of the same age.
- Calculate drug dosages with care.
- Absorption in the stomach is different in children under 2 years of age.
- Report all ADRs and suspected ADRs using yellow card scheme.
- Do not add the drug to the child's feed (there may be an interaction or the child may not complete their feed).
- Children may require higher doses than adults because they have higher metabolic rates.
- Where possible follow manufacturer's instructions as to frequency and duration of administration of medicines especially in the case of potentially toxic drugs.

    Adverse drug reactions (ADRs).

Calculating drug dosages in children

Doses are generally calculated using the child's body weight in kilograms.

Age ranges for calculating drug doses

- First month (neonates).
- Up to a year of age (infants).
- 1–5 years.
- 6–12 years (BNF latest version).

NB: with obese children, calculate dosage on the basis of ideal height and weight for age. Greater accuracy in drug calculation can be achieved using body surface area.

Formula to calculate surface area =

Surface area of patient (m^2) x adult dose/1.8

Formula to calculate drug dosage =

(What you want/what you've got) x what it's in

Example (required dose/actual dose) x dilution

Drug A contains 500mg in 5ml. To give 600mg:

600mg/500 x 5= 6mls

Consent
📖 Prescribing and the law.

Concordance
Where appropriate (depending on the child's age and your assessment of their competency) involve the parent/carer.

Writing the prescription
- Follow the guidelines in the BNF (latest edition).[1]
- It is a legal requirement to write the child's age if prescribing for children less than 12 years old.
- It is preferable to state the child's age for all prescriptions for children.
- Always state the strengths and formulation of the medication e.g capsules or tablets.
📖 Writing a prescription.

Advice for parents
- Do not dilute the drug in the child's milk/water nor add to the child's food unless you are instructed to do so by the prescriber. Diluting the drug may lead to the child getting the suboptimal dose if he/she does not complete the feed. Some drugs may interact with food or milk.
- Dispense the medicine using the device you have been provided with e.g. a syringe or spoon.
- Keep all medicines out of the reach of children.

NB: all drugs for children must be dispensed in a re-closable, child-resistant container.

Prescribing for rare conditions
For prescribing for rare paediatric conditions see 'Prescribing for children' in the current edition of the BNF.[1]

1 BNF for Children (latest edition) London. British Medical Association and Royal Pharmaceutical Society of Great Britain, London. http://bnfc.org
2 Kelly, J. (2000). Adverse Drug Effects; a nursing concern. Whurr, London.

Licensing

Many medicines essential for treating childhood conditions are not licensed for use in children.

- Unlicensed medication can be prescribed by a supplementary prescriber as part of a CMP.
- A supplementary prescriber can also prescribe medication which is outside of product licence as part of an agreed CMP.

📖 Breastfeeding and prescribing

Prescribing for people with renal disease

Considerations

Prescribing for people with renal impairment requires careful consideration as metabolism of the drug may be altered.

- Drugs and their metabolites may not be excreted quickly enough to avoid toxicity, e.g. opioids and some antibiotics.
- Renal impairment may be made worse. For example, patients with mild renal failure (see below) who are prescribed non-steroidal anti-inflammatory drugs (NSAIDs) may suffer increased sodium and water retention and further deterioration of renal function.
- Some drugs (potassium sparing diuretics, ACE inhibitors, and NSAIDs for example) may cause hyperkalemia.
- Sensitivity to some drugs may be increased.
- Side effects are tolerated poorly by patients in renal failure.
- Reduction of renal function may affect the efficacy of some drugs.
- Older people often have a degree of renal impairment.[1]

Grades of renal failure

For prescribing purposes, renal failure is subjectively divided into three grades:

- In **mild renal failure** the patient has a glomerula filtration rate (GFR) of 20–50 ml/minute and a serum creatinine of 150–300 µmol/litre.
- In **moderate renal failure** the patient has a GFR of 10–20 ml/minute and a serum creatinine of 300–700 µmol/litre.
- In **severe renal failure** the patient has a GFR of less than 10 ml/minute and a serum creatinine of greater than 700 µmol/litre.

> **Normal values:**
>
> GFR: 100 ml/minute
> Creatinine: 70–150 µmol/litre

See current BNF for a table of drugs to be avoided or used with caution in renal impairment.

📖 Prescribing for older people.

Further reading

Bardsley, A. (2003). Urinary tract infections: prevention and treatment of a common problem. *Nurse Prescribing*, 1(3).

Begg, E. J. (2003). *Instant clinical pharmacology*. Blackwell Publishing, Oxford.

Dunning, T. (2003) *Care of people with diabetes* (2nd edn). Blackwell Publishing, Oxford.

O'Callaghan, C., Brenner, M. (2000). *The Kidney at a glance*. Blackwell science, Oxford.

Thomas, N. (ed.) (2004). *Advanced renal care*. Blackwell Publishing, Oxford. Smith, T., Thomas, N. (2002). Renal Nursing. Ballière and Tindall, London.

---

1 Department of Health (1998). *Health Survey for England. vol 1: Findings*. The Stationary Office, London. In: DoH (2001). *Medicines and Older people*. NSF, The Stationary Office, London. http://www.doh.gov.uk/nsf/medicinesop

Prescribing in pregnancy

Risk versus benefit

When considering whether to prescribe for a pregnant woman, the prescriber must always consider the risk versus benefit ratio.

Safe practice

- Only prescribe for pregnant women when it is essential.
- Counsel the mother on the risk versus benefit of prescribing.
- Where possible, avoid prescribing for pregnant women during the first trimester.
- Prescribe drugs which have been tried and tested as safe in pregnancy.

Teratogenic effects (harm to the fetus)

Drugs can harm the fetus throughout the gestational period. Because of the obvious risks, there is very little experimental research data on prescribing for pregnant women.

First trimester

The greatest risk of the occurrence of congenital malformation is during the first semester and between 3–11 weeks. When possible, avoid prescribing during this period.

Second and third trimesters

Drugs administered to the mother at these stages may have toxic effects on fetal tissue and may affect fetal growth.

Immediately before and during labour

Drugs administered to the mother at this time may adversely affect the fetus and may have an effect on the duration and outcome of labour. They may also affect the new born baby.

Poisoning and chemical exposures in pregnancy 0870 600 6266 (24-hour service).

Drugs which are easily transported across the placenta include

- Narcotics
- Steroids
- Antibiotics
- Anaesthetics.

Risks versus benefits of prescribing for epilepsy

- Anti-convulsants can cause congenital abnormalities.[2]
- Convulsions can cause fetal mortality or morbidity. To manage epilepsy in pregnancy, give the lowest effective dose and monitor drug levels closely.

Appendix 4 in the latest edition of the BNF[1] provides an up to date table of which drugs should be avoided at which trimester during pregnancy.

1 British Medical Association and Royal Pharmaceutical Society of Great Britain. *British National Formulary* (latest edn). BMA, London.
2 McManus Kuller, J. (1990). Effects on the fetus and newborn of medications commonly used during pregnancy. *Journal of Perinatal Neonatal Nursing*, **3**, 73–87. cited in: J Kelly (2000). *Adverse Drug Effects: A Nursing Concern*. Whurr, London

Breastfeeding and prescribing

When considering prescribing for women who are breastfeeding remember that generally the advantages of breastfeeding outweigh the disadvantages. The risk–benefit ratio to the infant needs to be carefully considered when administering drugs to breastfeeding mothers. However, as drugs are only secreted into breast milk in small volumes, the benefits of breastfeeding generally outweigh the risks to the infant. Women should be advised to take drugs only if necessary; where possible, drug therapy should be delayed until the mother has completed breastfeeding. Always use the prescribing pyramid and apply the principles of good prescribing.[1] For breastfeeding clients, recommend or prescribe medication for necessity only.

- Consider the patient.
- Is it appropriate to prescribe?
- Can you give lifestyle/health promotion advice instead?
- If not, consider the product
  - Is it safe?
  - Is it indicated for use for breastfeeding women?
  - Is it cautioned for use when breastfeeding?
- Remember to ask the client about any over the counter drugs she may be taking.

For interactions and cautions and contraindications see Appendix 5 in the BNF (latest edition).[2]

- Many drugs are lipid soluble. The amount of drug which is secreted in the breast milk is therefore dependant to a greater or lesser extent on its lipid solubility.
- However, in many cases only small amounts of the drug are excreted in breast milk.
- Very few drugs are licensed for prescribing for breastfeeding.
- Remember that in some cases it is essential for the parent to continue with medication e.g. prescribing for epilepsy, depression, and many chronic diseases.
- Some medication dosage may need to be adjusted to account for breastfeeding women.

Prescribing for mild to moderate pain while breastfeeding

Paracetamol is the drug of choice for mild to moderate pain. Some analgesic drugs pass less easily into breast milk than others. For instance, in the case of simple analgesia it is advisable for the breastfeeding mother to take paracetamol rather than aspirin. Aspirin can pass into breast milk and into the breastfeeding infant causing a risk of Reye's syndrome in the baby.

---

1 National Prescribing Centre (1999). The Principles of Prescribing. *Nurse Prescribing Bulletin* Number 1. NPC Liverpool.
2 British Medical Association and Royal Pharmaceutical Society of Great Britain. *British National Formulary.* (latest edn). BMA, London.

Route of administration

- Drugs which do not undergo first-pass metabolism (intravenous drugs) pass to the infant in higher concentrations.
- Inhaled drugs have less tendency to pass into breast milk than oral drugs.

Volume of breast milk/drug concentration

- Production of breast milk is stimulated as a response to infant feeding.
- The concentration and amount of drug which is consumed by the infant is proportional to the volume of the baby's feed.

Time of administration

- It is advisable to take drugs immediately after feeding in order to maximize the length of time between taking the drug and the next feed.
- Drugs to be taken only once a day can be taken before the baby's longest sleep time.

Maturity of infant

- The baby has normal renal clearance by 3 days after birth.
- The maturation rate of liver enzymes can vary and some may take up to 1 year to mature.
- Caution needs to be exercised when administering drugs to the mother which are liver enzyme inducers or liver enzyme inhibitors.

Molecular density/molecular weight

- Drugs with a high molecular weight and large plasma proteins can pass into breast milk for up to one week after birth.
- After one week only drugs with a low molecular weight can pass into breast milk.
- Drugs with a high molecular weight include heparin and insulin.

Plasma protein binding

- Plasma proteins which bind to drugs only pass into the breast milk in small amounts.
- Phenytoin is highly plasma protein bound.

Lipid solubility

- Drugs which are lipid soluble pass easily into breast milk.
- Diazepam is highly lipid soluble.

pH

- The pH of breast milk is 7.2 (neutral).
- Drugs with weak bases (slightly alkaline) have increased lipid solubility and pass more easily into breast milk.
- Drugs with weak bases include erythromycin and antihistamines.
- Weak bases can become ionized by an acid PH leading to increased concentration of such drugs in the breast milk.

📖 Prescribing for children.

Further reading

Banta-Wright, S.A. (1997). Minimising Infant exposure to and risks from Medications while breastfeeding. *Journal of Perinatal and Neonatal Nursing* 11, 71–4. Cited in: J Kelly (2000) *Adverse Drug Effects: A Nursing Concern*, p. 82. Whurr London.

Chapter 12

Medical conditions

Prescribing for musculoskeletal conditions

Brief anatomy and physiology of the musculoskeletal structure

The musculoskeletal structure comprises:
- bones
- muscles
- joints.

Bones
Functions
- Provide framework for protection of the internal organs of the body.
- Enable movement.
- Store minerals and salts.

Structure
- 30% water.
- Soft and flexible.
- Three layers
  - Hard outer shell—compact bone, comprised of tiny cylindrical units called the Haversian system.
  - Haversian system—provides strength as each cylinder lies orientated to the greatest stress for the bone, i.e. lies lengthways in the shaft of the femur.
  - Inner—spongy, trabecular, or cancellous bone.
  - Bone marrow—soft jellylike substance that lies centrally.
- Blood supply to bring nutrients.
- Nerve supply to enable sensory detection.

Skeletal muscles (striped/striated)
Functions
- Work in pairs one either side of a bone to facilitate movement.
- Work in groups, some relaxing, some contracting, to take the strain of complex movements, maintenance of position and body posture.

Structure
- Over 600 in the body.
- Arranged in bundles with the cells forming a striped pattern.
- Under conscious control—voluntary muscles.

Joints
Functions
- Provide a framework.
- Provide an interface between two bones.

Structure
- Bones are linked to each other by ligaments to form a joint.
- Can be fibrous (skull), cartilaginous (vertebrae), or synovial (knee).

Movement

This is achieved through a series of levers. A lever is a way of moving a load by the application of pressure. The body has three main types of lever:

First order lever (e.g. moving the head)

Here the fulcrum (pivoting point) of the lever is positioned between the load (skull and contents) and the effort (the muscular contractions/relaxations of the neck muscles).

Second order lever (e.g. standing on tiptoe)

Here the load (the body) is placed between the fulcrum and the effort (calf and foot muscle activity).

Third order lever (e.g. bending the elbow)

Here three-way effort (forearm muscular activity) is between the load (the hand and contents) and the fulcrum.

Soft tissue injuries

Sprains

Definition
Overstretching and tearing of ligaments varying in severity from minor sparse fibrous tears to disruption of a complete ligament complex.

Signs and symptoms
- Pain
- Tenderness
- Soft tissue swelling.

Treatment of minor sprains
- Ice.
- Elevate.
- Compression with an elastic support or strapping.
- Progressive mobilization as symptoms allow.
- Pain relief.

If a sprain has caused a complete rupture of the ligaments associated with joint instability, surgery may be indicated.

Strains

Definition
Grade 1 and 2 strains involve torn muscle fibres but intact muscle sheaths. Grade 3 involves a partial rupture of the muscle sheath and Grade 4 is a complete muscle rupture.

Signs and symptoms
As sprains.

Treatment
- Grades 1 and 2 as sprains.
- Grades 3 and 4 may require surgery.

Minor contusions

Definition
Superficial ecchymoses, soft tissue swelling and localized pain caused by a direct impact.

Signs and symptoms
As sprains.

Treatment
- Ice
- Analgesia
- Early mobilization.

Haematoma

Definition

An accumulation of blood resulting from a traumatic disruption of vascular structures within bone, muscle, or soft tissues.

Signs and symptoms

As sprains.

Treatment

- Compression dressings
- Ice
- Massage.

Skeletal muscular spasm in palliative care

Definition
A muscle spasm of long or short duration. These may arise in muscles close to bone metastasis, be drug induced, or caused by damage to nerve pathways.

Signs and symptoms
Painful and prolonged involuntary muscle contraction.

Treatment
- Skeletal muscle relaxants
- Massage
- Relaxation techniques.

📖 Basic principles of pharmacology.
📖 History taking.
📖 Physical examination.

Table 12.1 Symptoms which may be significant of more serious conditions

Symptom	Possible diagnosis
Difficulty in passing urine	Cauda equine syndrome
Loss of anal sphincter tone	
Faecal incontinence	
Numbness around the anus, perineum, or genitalia	
Severe, prolonged motor weakness	
Unilateral leg pain which is more severe than the back pain	Nerve root pain
Pain radiates to the foot and toes	
Pain is accompanied by numbness and parathesia	
Pain is reduced by straight leg raising, reflex, and sensory changes	

Acute uncomplicated low back pain

Definition
Pain experienced in the back involving the lumbar, lumbar sacral and sacroiliac areas.

Causes assessment
Strain to the muscles or tendons caused by overuse or abnormal stress and exercise.

Assessment
- History .
- Age.
- Sex.
- Medical conditions.
- Employment.
- Exact nature of any injury.
- Duration, position, and type of pain—is it radiating?
- Any unaccustomed activity?
- Has the patient had this before?
- If so when, and how often?
- What have they taken in the past which has worked?
- Have they tried anything today?
- What is the impact of the symptoms?
- Stress.
- Other symptoms.

Signs and symptoms
- Patient generally between the ages of 20–55 years.
- Pain in the lumbosacral region, buttocks, and thighs.
- Pain of a mechanical type.

Treatment
- Pain relief. Analgesia and/or NSAIDs.
- Advise to keep to normal activity.
- If symptoms are severe prescribe muscle relaxants.
- To seek advice if limb numbness or weakness, or if any new bladder or bowel problems occur.

📖 Basic principles of pharmacology.
📖 History taking.
📖 Physical examination.

Acute uncomplicated neck pain

Definition signs and symptoms

Pain caused by a sprain or persistent twisting of the neck.

Causes

Neck hyperextension as in whiplash.

History

- Any injury?
- When?
- Any visual disturbances?
- Any dizziness or tinnitus?
- Vertigo?
- Headache?
- Backache?
- Altered sensation?
- Lack of power?

Signs and symptoms

- Neck pain
- Stiffness.

Treatment

As for uncomplicated back pain.

📖 Basic principles of pharmacology.
📖 History taking.
📖 Physical examination.

Prescribing for the circulatory system

A brief anatomy and physiology of the circulatory system

Blood flows around the body through a series of veins, venules, arteries, arterioles, and capillaries.

The system comprises two circuits:

Systemic circulation

From the heart around the body via arteries and back to the heart via veins.

Pulmonary circulation

From the right ventricle of the heart into the lungs and back into the heart via the right atrium.

Veins

- Return deoxygenated blood to the right atrium of the heart.
- Contain approx ¾ of total blood volume.
- Take blood from the capillaries back to the heart.

Arteries

- Carry oxygenated blood away from the heart.
- Branch 15–20 times reducing in size.
- Contain $^1/_5$ of the blood volume.

Arterioles

- Small arteries are called arterioles.
- Arterioles lead into capillaries.

Capillaries

- Carry blood from the arterioles to the venules, facilitating the passage of oxygen and nutrients to surrounding tissues.
- Contain $^1/_{20}$ of the blood volume.
- Walls comprise a single layer of endothelial cells.

The walls of arteries and veins are comprised of three layers specific to their function. See Table 12.2.

Table 12.2 Structure of the blood veins and arteries

Name	Structure	Function
Tunica adventia	Outermost layer of vessel	Stability
	Generally thicker in veins than tunica media	Anchorage
	Forms a connective tissue sheath	
Tunica media	Involuntary muscle, stimulated by involuntary nerve fibres	Alteration of lumen size
	Elastic fibres	
Tunica intima	Smooth endothelial cells	Lining and formation of valves and basement membrane

Venous system

Input mechanisms to enable the return of venous blood to the heart.
- Respiratory pump
- Venous pump
- Venous valves.

Respiratory pump

On inhalation:
- The thoracic cavity expands.
- ↓p in the pleural cavities.
- Air is pulled into the lungs.
- Simultaneously blood flow from the small veins in the abdominal cavity and lower body into the inferior vena cava and right atrium.

On exhalation:
- Thoracic cavity decreases in size.
- ↑p.
- Air is forced out of the lungs.
- Venous blood forced into the right atrium.

Venous pump

Venous system of the leg comprises:
- femoral, popliteal, and tibial deep veins.
- each are encased in a tough, muscle sheath.
- long and short saphenous superficial are outside this sheath.
- short perforator veins connect through the sheath.

The pump works by:
- weight of blood in the leg veins exert ↑p up to 90mmHg in the foot when standing still.
- this ↑p is lower than that in the veins and capillaries.
- when standing and walking the calf muscles first contract becoming shorter and thicker.
- compressing nearby blood vessels move blood up towards the heart.
- calf muscles then relax allowing vessels to fill again.
- blood pools in the lower leg if standing still for a long time.

Venous valves

Semi-lunar folds of endothelial tissue form the valves present in the leg veins:
- the valves point in the direction of blood flow.
- allow blood to flow in one direction only.
- prevent it from flowing back to the capillaries.
- this compartmentalizes the vein dividing the weight of blood evenly in the vein. Blood is then squeezed back towards the heart by the movement of skeletal muscle.
- perforator connecting veins are important in this process.

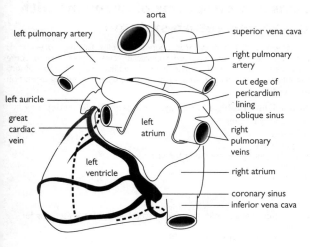

Fig. 12.1 The venous drainage of the heart—posterior view of heart.

Signs and symptoms of problems with the venous return system

If the valves in the perforator connecting veins fail, high pressure is passed to weaker unsupported superficial veins. These then become distended and tortuous (varicose veins). If capillary ↑p fluid is forced into the interstitial spaces, oedema, pigmentation, eczema, and leg ulceration may follow.

Superficial phlebitis (inflammation of the vein walls)

Signs and symptoms

- Redness
- Tenderness
- Swelling along the course of the vein
- Fever
- Lymphangitis.

Treatment

- Heat
- Non-steroidal anti-inflammatory drugs (NSAIDs) 📖 Prescribing for pain
- Compression stockings.

Causes

Usually follows an injury to a vein followed by an inflammatory response.

Complications

Phlebitis can lead to venous thrombosis (a clot).

Compression therapy

- Graduated pressure from toe to base of knee.
- Pressure highest at the ankle.
- Pressure lowest at the knee.

Compression hosiery is one way of achieving this.

- Below knee or thigh length socks, stockings or tights which conform to the BSI made-to-measure standard sizes.
- Stockings are classified according to pressure exerted at the ankle and the gradients at knee and thigh.

Types of hosiery

- Circular knit: nylon and cotton yarn—poor stretch.
- Flat bed knit: cotton, nylon and nylon plated—greater stretch.
- Net stockings: seamed net fabric.
- One way stretch: class I only.

Table 12.3 Classes of compression hosiery

Class	Description of support	Pressure	Indications
Class I	Light Mild	14–17mmHg at the ankle ≤80% of ankle pressure at calf ≤85% of calf pressure at mid thigh	Superficial varices For use during pregnancy
Class II	Medium Moderate	18–24mmHg at the ankle ≤70% of ankle pressure at calf ≤70% of calf pressure at mid thigh	Medium severe varices Ulcer treatment Prevention of recurrence Mild oedema During pregnancy
Class III	Strong	25–35mmHg at the ankle ≤70% of ankle pressure at calf ≤70% of calf pressure at mid thigh	Gross varices Post-thrombotic venous insufficiency Gross oedema Ulcer treatment Prevention of recurrence

Selection of compression hosiery

- Patient's age
- Dexterity or disability
- Skin condition
- Appearance of hosiery
- Type usually worn by patient (tights or stockings).

Measurement points for compression hosiery

Circumference

(1) Top of thigh
(2) Mid point between 1 and 3
(3) Knee at widest point
(4) Base of knee
(5) Widest calf circumference
(6) Mid point between 5 and 7
(7) Ankle at narrowest point (2–4 cms above ankle bone)
(8) Widest point on foot for stocking to pass over
(9) Toe base.

Length

(1) Draw around patient's foot whilst they are standing on a piece of paper
(2) Toe to back of heel
(3) Measurement between each of 9 points above.

Fitting
- Turn stocking inside out at heel
- Pull up two handed with thumbs inserted in either side
- Check heel in correct position
- Ease up over the leg
- Check there are no ridges or tight bands
- Take off at night and apply first thing in the morning
- Patients may need to wear for a short time only to start with
- If the hosiery is effective in reducing oedema re-measure and prescribe
- If unable to tolerate Class III then two pairs of Class I worn at the same time may be tolerated.[1] Pressure is cumulative.

Advice on washing hosiery
- Handwash at 40°C.
- Frequent washing improves shape.
- Should provide pressure for 3–4 months.

Points to consider when prescribing
- The quantity—single or pair?
- Article/style/type and any accessories.
- Compression Class I, II, or III.
- Patient's measurements, if made to measure are required.
- Issues of concordance—no point prescribing if not going to be worn.

Contraindications
- Severe arteriosclerosis or other ischemic vascular disease.
- Skin lesions, allergies, or gangrene.
- Recent vein ligation.

1 Fentem, P. H. (1986). Elastic hosiery. *Pharmacy Update*, **5**, 200–5.

Haemorrhoids (piles)

Definition
Varices in the veins of the anorectal canal.

Causes
- Elevated venous pressure causes these vessels to stretch and dilate.
- Commonly, straining to pass a stool when constipated.
- Pregnancy.

Classification and signs and symptoms
- Bleeding—blood on stool around the toilet pan.
- Temporarily or permanently prolapsed—blue-coloured, localized swellings in the perianal region.
- Thrombosed – perianal pain[1].

Advice
- Avoid constipation and straining.
- Information on high fibre and fluid intake.

Non-surgical treatment
Suppositories and ointments
- Hancock[2] suggests these have little more than a placebo effect.
- Should not be used for more than 7 days.

Corticosteroids combined with local anaesthetic
📖 Skin regarding topical corticosteroids.

1 Travis, S.P.L., Taylor, R.H., Misiewicz, J. J. (1998). *Gastroenterology* (2nd edn). Blackwell Science, Oxford.
2 Hancock, B. D. (1999). Hemorrhoids. In D. J. Jones (ed) *ABC of Colorectal disease* (2nd edn). BMJ, London.

Prescribing for the ear

Brief anatomy and physiology of the ear

Structure of the ear

Three main parts: external ear, middle ear, and inner ear (see Fig. 12.2).

External ear

- Pinna: a skin-covered flap which protects and channels sound waves into the external auditory meatus.
- External auditory meatus: about 2.5 cm long in the adult and protected by fine hairs and wax-secreting ceruminous glands.
- Function of these secretions and hairs is to prevent airborne particles from reaching the inner ear canal.
- With pH 6.0, the cerumen (earwax) provides a defence against microorganisms.
- This area ends at the tympanic membrane.

Middle ear

- The thin, transparent tympanic membrane stretches across the entrance to the middle ear vibrating when moved by sound.
- The air-filled middle ear, facilitated by the auditory ossicles (the malleus, incus, and stapes), transports these vibrations to the fluid-filled inner ear.
- The barrier between the middle and inner ear is the oval window to which the stapes is attached.
- Movements of the stapes cause the oval window to bow and flex, facilitating transference of vibrations into the inner ear.

Inner ear

Vibrations transported through the inner ear are interpreted and perceived as sounds by the central nervous system (CNS).

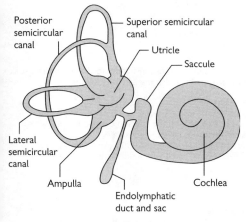

Fig. 12.2 Diagram of the inner ear

Drugs for the ear

- Astringent preparations
- Anti-inflammatory preparations
- Anti-infective preparations
- Ear wax softeners.

These may be in the form of ear drops instilled into the ear or as a soak on a piece of ribbon gauze with which the ear is packed.

Ear drops

- Warm to body heat prior to instillation.
- Encourage the patient to lie with the affected ear uppermost for 5–10 minutes after the drops have been instilled.
- Do not prescribe to patients with a history of ear disease, those complaining of dizziness, or those with a discharge form the ear.

Assessment

History

Difficulty with hearing

- Duration of the problem.
- Onset of the problem—was it gradual or sudden?
- Previous history.
- Any trauma.

Routine physical examination
Look for:

- foreign bodies
- reported irritation or itching
- infection
- build-up of wax
- scaliness
- narrowing of the ear canal because of swelling
- redness
- pain
- discharge
- hearing loss.

Common conditions

See the current BNF[1] for a list of conditions for which the nurse prescriber can prescribe.

Conductive hearing loss

Definition
Difficulty in hearing as sound waves are not transferred to the inner ear.

Prevention
Earwax is a normal secretion; warn patients to avoid impacting the wax by using implements such as hairpins and matchsticks as probes.

Causes
- Most common cause is a build-up of earwax.
- Blockage of the outer ear by foreign body.
- Infection of the inner ear.
- Perforation of the tympanic membrane.
- Immobilization of one or all of the auditory ossicles.

Signs and symptoms
Hearing loss.

Treatment
- Instil drops, i.e. almond or olive oil ear drops (ceruminolytics) to soften the wax.
- If ear syringing is required following softening of the wax, it should be undertaken by a practitioner who is proficient in the technique.

Otitis externa

Definition
- Inflammation of the outer ear.
- Affecting the pinna and/or external auditory meatus.
- It may vary in severity from mild to severe.

Causes
- Infection: bacterial mostly and sometimes secondary fungal infections.
- Reaction to materials found in earrings or earphones (contact dermatitis).

Signs and symptoms
- Scaliness
- Narrowing of the ear canal because of swelling
- Redness
- Pain
- Discharge
- Hearing loss.

---

1 British Medical Association and Royal Pharmaceutical Society of Great Britain. *British National Formulary*. (latest edn). BMA, London.

Treatment
- Clean and remove any debris or discharge; this is often enough.
- If infection, then prescribe a topical antibiotic and analgesia.

Prescribing for the eye

Prescribing for the eye

Brief anatomy and physiology of the eye

Assessment of the condition of the eye rests on an understanding of the of the normal protective functions and a history of the duration of the presenting condition.

Structure of the eye

Eyelids (palpebrae)

- Epithelial tissue.
- Function is to protect the eye by keeping the surface clear and lubricated.
- Lubrication provided by a lipid-rich secretion of the meibomian glands (modified sebaceous glands) and the lachrymal caruncle.
- Eyelashes prevent contamination of the eye.
- The conjunctiva covers the inner surface of the eye (palpebral conjunctiva), the outer surface of the eyeball (bulbar conjunctiva), and the cornea.

Eyeball (see Fig. 12.3)

Kept moist and clean by secretions of the accessory glands and goblet cells.

Administration of drugs for the eye

Eye drops

- Penetrate the globe, probably through the cornea.
- Some systemic absorption follows instillation into the eye, but this is variable and often undesirable.
- Usually instilled into the pocket formed by pulling forward the lower lid.
- The eye should be kept closed for as long as possible to allow absorption.
- Eye-drop dispensers are for repeated use by individual patients.

Eye ointments

- A small amount of ointment is smeared along the inside of the lower lid.
- Blinking helps to spread the melted ointment.

Eye lotions

- Flush out foreign bodies from the conjunctival sack.
- Used for first-aid treatment.

When more than one product is being used to treat the eye, it is advisable to leave 5 min or so between instillations.

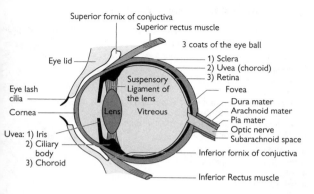

Assessment of the eye

History

- Duration of the problem.
- Onset of the problem—was it gradual or sudden?
- Full medical history.
- Any trauma.

Routine physical examination

Look for:
- redness
- discharge
- foreign bodies
- reported irritation or itching of the eyelid margins
- gritty sensation
- stye (chalazion)
- scales attached to the eyelids
- appearance of the sclera (cobblestone appearance of the lining of the upper lid may indicate allergic conjunctivitis)
- feeling of a foreign body in the eye
- visual aquity
- pupil size and reaction.

📖 Clinical and physical examination.
📖 History taking.

Common conditions of the eye

See the current BNF[1] for a list of conditions for which the nurse prescriber can prescribe.

Blepharitis
Definition
- Inflammation of the eyelid margins.
- Two main types:
  - staphylococcal, caused by either *Staphylococcus aureus* or *Staphylococcus epidermidis*; or
  - seborrhoeic, associated with *Pityrosporum ovale*.
- Often found in combination.

Signs and symptoms
- Soreness of the eyelids
- Irritation
- Itching of the eyelid margins
- Gritty sensation
- Stye
- Scales on the lower lid margins and lashes.

Treatment
- Keep lids clean: patients may need instruction on how to clean the eye and apply ointment.
- Treat any infection with antibiotic ointment usually 3–4 times daily.
- Topical eye treatments may cause transient blurring of vision or stinging pain; warn patients of these possibilities.
- If eyes dry, keep moist with artificial tears.
- Severe cases may need oral antibiotics.
- Prevent inflammation returning by continuing to treat for 1 month after the cessation of symptoms.

Conjunctivitis
Definition
- Inflammation of the conjunctiva of the eye.
- Sometimes called 'red eye'.
- Most common eye condition in the world.
- Causative agent can be either allergic or infective.

Allergic conjunctivitis
Causes
- Often associated with allergic reactions such as asthma and hay fever (allergic rhinitis).
- Sometimes as a result of contact with chemicals such as eye make-up.
- Use of contact lenses.

1 British Medical Association and Royal Pharmaceutical Society of Great Britain. *British National Formulary* (latest edn). BMA, London.

Signs and symptoms

- Itching.
- Redness.
- Oedematous clear discharge.
- 'Cobblestone' appearance inside the upper lid due to oedema.
- Feeling of a foreign body in the eye.
- Visual acuity is normal.
- Pupils react normally.

Treatment

- Apply topical antihistamines or mast cell stabilizers.
- Instruct patients on how to clean the eye and apply ointment or drops.
- Warn patients that eye treatments may cause transient blurring of vision or stinging pain.
- Oral antihistamines may be necessary.
- Topical corticosteroids may be resorted to, but there is a risk of steroid-induced cataracts and glaucoma with these.
- Soft contact lenses should not be worn during treatment with eye drops as they may absorb either the active medication or preservatives within it.

Infective conjunctivitis

Causes

- Infection may be viral or bacterial.
- Bacterial infection most commonly due to *Staphylococcus* strains
- Viral infection is more common than bacterial, usually due to one of the adenoviruses.
- Viral infections usually occur in epidemics.

Bacterial conjunctivitis

Causes

- Commonly due to *Staphylococcus*.
- Followed by infection by *Streptococcus pneumoniae* and/or *Haemophilus influenzae*.

Signs and symptoms

- Purulent exudates (idicative of bacterial infections).
- Sticky eyelids on waking.
- Usually starts in one eye and is spread by the patient's hands or fomites to the other.
- It spreads from person to person in this way.
- Feeling of a foreign body in the eye.
- Visual acuity is normal.
- Pupils react normally.

Treatment

- Apply topical antibiotics, usually one drop every 2 hrs initially, with the timing between drops extended as the infection abates.
- Continue eye drops for up to 48 hrs after the infection is controlled.

- Eye ointment is usually applied at night and eye drops during the day; however, if ointment is used alone, then it should be applied 3–4 times a day.
- Instruct the patient on how to clean the eye and apply ointment or drops.
- Warn patients that eye treatments may cause transient blurring of vision or stinging pain.

Prevention
- Strict hygiene measures are required to prevent the spread from one eye to the other and from person to person.
- Advise patients:
  - to use their own pillowcase, flannel, and towel
  - to administer their own drops and ointment where possible
  - to wash their hands before and after touching the eyes
  - to always clean an uninfected eye first then move to the infected eye
  - not to wear contact lenses
  - to avoid eye make-up.

Viral conjunctivitis
Causes
- More common than bacterial conjunctivitis.
- Commonly caused by adenoviruses.
- Some viral serotypes may cause severe keratoconjunctivitis.

Signs and symptoms
- Eyes feel gritty.
- Watery discharge (indicative of viral infections).
- Feeling of a foreign body in the eye.
- VA is normal.
- Pupils react normally.
- Sometimes associated with sore throat, upper respiratory tract infection, and fever.
- May persist for weeks—a longer duration than bacterial conjunctivitis.
- Severe keratoconjunctivitis may have lasting visual disturbances, photophobia, and discomfort.

Treatment
- Apply topical antibiotics to prevent secondary bacterial infection.
- As for bacterial infection, see above.

Prevention
As for bacterial conjunctivitis, see above.

Acute glaucoma
This occurs when the drainage system of the eye becomes blocked allowing fluid to build up resulting in an increase in intra-ocular pressure. If untreated this condition will lead to blindness.

Early symptoms such as sub-acute angle glaucoma may occur. The patient is aware of halos around lights at night accompanied by an aching in the eye and blurring of vision.

Further reading

More information regarding glaucoma:

🖳 www.fightingblindness/i.e._FB_EC_glaucoma.htm
🖳 www.merck.com/mrkshared/mmanual/section8/chapter100/100c.jsp

Prescribing for problems within the endocrine system

Prescribed items for the management of diabetes mellitus

Diabetes mellitus is a chronic and progressive disease which alters the body's management of carbohydrate and fat metabolism. It is divided into type 1 diabetes (previously known as insulin-dependant diabetes mellitus IDDM) in which there is an absence of insulin, and type 2 diabetes which is caused by the body's inefficient use of endogenous insulin (insulin resistance) and/or insufficient production of insulin.

It can affect:
• All ages and races.
• Poor people in affluent societies and people of South Asian, African, and African-Caribbean descent are particularly at risk.

Diabetes impacts on both physical and psychological health.
• Physical long-term complications can lead to both micro and macro vascular disease including stroke, heart disease, amputation, renal failure, neuropathy, and blindness.
• Diabetes through restricted job choices, driving restrictions and the decisions of financial institutions can affect the material well-being of both individuals with the disease and their families.

Type 1 diabetes

Type 1 diabetes is usually diagnosed in children, teenagers, and young adults. It is caused because the β cells (insulin-producing cells) in the pancreas have been destroyed by the body's autoimmune system.

Drugs used to treat type 1 diabetes
- Insulin (see Table 12.4 for different types)
- Glucogon hypo kit
- Hypostop gel.

Other prescribable items
- Hypodermic equipment
- Pen injectors (check these are compatible with insulin cartridge prescribed)
- Needles
- Syringes
- Finger prickers and lancets
- Needle clippers
- Blood glucose monitoring equipment
- Ketone monitoring blood and urine testing sticks.

Table 12.4 Insulin types and actions
N.B. all timings are approximate and vary from preparation to preparation.

Type of insulin	Name	Onset	Peak	Duration
Rapid acting insulin analogues	Insulin lispro	5–10 mins	30–90 mins	3–5 hrs
	Insulin aspart	10–20 mins	1–3 hours	3–5 hrs
Short acting N.B. pork and beef insulins work more slowly	Soluble	30 mins	1–4 hrs	12 hrs
Intermediate and long acting	Insulin glargine	–	–	24 hrs
	Insulin zinc suspension	1–3 hrs	7–16hrs	23–30 hrs
	Insulin zinc suspension (crystalline)	4–8hrs	8–24hrs	24–28 hrs
	Isophane	30 mins–2hrs	1–12 hrs	11–24 hrs
	Protamine zinc suspension	4–6 hrs	10–20 hrs	25–35 hrs
Biphasic	Biphasic insulin aspart	–	8 hrs	13 hrs
	Biphasic insulin lispro	–	8hrs	13 hrs
	Biphasic Isophane insulin	5–15 mins	depending on mix	20–24 hrs

Type 2 diabetes

Type 2 diabetes is usually diagnosed in adults over the age of 40 years, although there has been an increase in the number of young people being diagnosed with the disease. People of South Asian decent are six times more likely to have type 2 diabetes and those of African or African-Caribbean decent are three times more likely to have the disease than members of the white population. The initial treatment for type 2 diabetes is a combination of increased exercise, diet and, if the patient is overweight, weight reduction. Most people with type 2 diabetes will progress to require oral hypoglycaemics and other antidiabetic drugs. Some may require a combination of oral hypoglycaemic drugs and insulin.

Drugs used to treat type 2 diabetes
Oral hypoglycaemics and antidiabetic preparations:
- Metformin
- Sulphonyureas
- Thiazolidinediones
- Alpha-glucosidase
- Insulin.

Medications to treat associated conditions
- Hypotensive medication
- Statins
- Nicotine replacement therapy
- Hypostop
- Anti-obesity medication/meal replacements (see National Obesity Forum guidelines on management of adult obesity in Primary Care www.nationalobesityforum.org.uk and NICE guidelines www.nice.org.uk).

Other products
- Blood and urine testing sticks for glucose and ketones
- Finger prickers and lancets
- Hypodermic devices (see above)
- Needle clippers.

All women with type 2 diabetes who become pregnant, must stop their oral hypoglycaemic drugs and will require insulin therapy during their pregnancy.

Gestational diabetes is experienced by some pregnant women who require insulin only during their pregnancy. This is often an indicator that they will be diagnosed with type 2 diabetes later in life.

Table 12.5 Examples of oral hypoglycaemics and antidiabetic drugs

Type and generic name	Action time	When taken
Biguanide (Metformin)	12 hours	2–3 times a day with or after food
Sulphonyureas		
Chlorpropamide	36–72 hrs	Once a day with food
Glibenclamide	16–24 hrs	Once a day with or immediately after the first meal of the day
Gliclazide	12–18 hrs	1 or 2 times a day with or shortly before food
Glimepiride	18–24hrs	Once a day shortly before the first meal
Glipizide	12–18 hrs	1–2 times a day before food
Tolbutamide	6–8 hrs	1–3 times a day with or immediately after food
Prandial glucose regulators		
Nateglinide	1–4hrs	Before each meal*
Repaglinide	1–6hrs	1–3 times a day with or immediately after food
Thiazolidinediones (glitizones) PPAR-γ agonist		
Pioglitizone		Once at the same time each day with or without food
Rosiglitazone		1–2 times at the same times each day with or without food
Rosiglitazone and metformin		Twice daily
Alpha glucosidase inhibitors (Acarbose)		Chewed with the first mouthful of each meal

* Nateglinide is intended to be taken with a meal – if the meal is missed the dose is missed.

Further reading

Department of Health (2001). *National Service Framework for diabetes: Standards.* DoH, London.
Department of Health (2003). *National Service Framework for diabetes: Delivery Strategy.* DoH, London.
NICE Guidelines.

Help

🔳 www.rcn.co.uk/diabetes resource

Thyroid hormones

These are used to treat:
- Hypothyroidism (myxoedema)
- Diffuse non-toxic goitre
- Hashimoto's thyroiditis (lymphadenoid goitre)
- Cancer of the thyroid.

Corticosteroids

In a healthy person the adrenal cortex secretes hydrocortisone (cortisol) which has a glucocorticoid (anti-inflammatory) activity and a weak mineralcorticoid activity. In addition, it secretes the mineral corticoid aldosterone.

Replacement therapy

In a deficiency of corticosteroids combination of both hydrocortisone and the mineralcorticoid fludrocortisone are prescribed. Following an adrenalectomy or in Addison's disease, hydrocortisone is prescribed. In acute adrenocortical insufficiency, hydrocortisone is given intravenously.

Glucocorticoid therapy

See current BNF for dose recommendations, indications, advantages, cautions, and contraindications.

Table 12.6 Thyroid hormones and antithyroid drugs

Condition	Medication
Hypothyroidism	**Thyroid hormones**
	Levothyroxine sodum/thyroxine sodium
Hyperthyroidism	**Antithyroid drugs**
	Carbimazole
	Iodine and iodide
	Propylthiouracil

Sex hormones

Female sex hormones

Oestrogens

These are required for:
- The secondary female sexual characteristics.
- The stimulation of myometrial hypertrophy.
- Endometrial hyperplasia.

Natural oestrogens are more appropriate for HRT (📖 HRT)
If long term therapy is needed, progesterone should be added to the oestrogen to reduce the risk of:
- Cystic hyperplasia of the endometrium as this may be a pre-cancerous state.
- Migraine or migraine like headaches.
- Diabetes (and the increased risk of CHD).
- Breast nodules.
- Breast cancer (if there is a family history with a first-degree relative).
- Increase in size of uterine fibroids.
- Exacerbation of the symptoms of endometriosis.

Progestogens

There are two groups of progestogens:
- Progesterone and its analogues
- Testosterone analogues.

Progestogens are used to treat:
- Endometriosis
- Menorrhagia
- Severe dysmenorrhoea.

They are also used for:
- Alleviation of premenstrual symptoms
- Prevention of spontaneous abortion for women with a history of recurrent miscarriage
- An oral contraceptive.

Male sex hormones and antagonists

Androgens

- In the healthy body, androgens inhibit pituitary gonadotrophin secretion, leading to the production of anabolic steroids and depression of spermatogenesis.
- They are required for masculinity and may be used as a replacement therapy for castrated adult males and those who are hypogonadal due to either pituitary or testicular disease.
- Depot IM injections of testosterone esters are the preferred preparations for replacement therapy.
- Implants of testosterone can be given to menopausal women as an adjunct to HRT in order to alleviate symptoms. Preparations are also available as patches, gel and for oral administration.

Anti-androgens

These may be used to treat severe hypersexuality and sexual deviation in the male. They inhibit spermatogenesis and result in reversible infertility.

Anabolic steroids

These can be used in the treatment of aplastic anaemia.

Other hormonal preparations and their uses

Anti-oestrogens

These may be used as a treatment for infertility in women who have oligomenorrhoea or secondary amenorrhea (associated with polycystic ovary disease).

By occupying the oestrogen receptors in the hypothalamus they interfere with feedback causing gonadotrophin release.

Anterior pituitary hormones

Corticotrophins

These are used to test adrenocortical function. If the plasma cortisol concentration fails to rise after their administration this is an indication of adrenocortical insufficiency.

Gonadotrophins

These are used in the treatment of infertility in women with proven hypopituitarism or those who have failed to conceive after receiving other infertility treatments. They have also been used to treat delayed puberty in young males.

Antidiuretic hormone antagonist

By blocking the renal tubule response to antidiuretic hormone this can be used to treat hyponatraemia.

Drugs affecting bone metabolism

Calcitonin

This hormone is involved with the parathyroid in the regulation of calcium balance and homeostasis in the body. It may be prescribed for post menopausal women who have osteoporosis.

It is used in severe Paget's disease for the relief of pain and some of the neurological symptoms. It is also used to lower plasma/calcium concentrations in patients with hypercalcaemia associated with cancer.

Bisphosphonates

These slow the rate of bone growth and dissolution thus reducing the rate of bone turnover.

They are used prophylactically for osteoporosis and are also used in the treatment of Paget's disease and hypercalcaemia associated with cancer.

Further reading

For further information and help please see the current BNF.

Links to journals, guidelines, patient handouts and research for endocrine disease are available from: ▣ http://omni.ac.uk

Prescribing for gastrointestinal problems

Anatomy and physiology of the gastrointestinal (GI) tract

See the list of conditions for which nurse prescribers are able to prescribe from the current CPF.

Many of the medications for treatment of the conditions included in this section are available as over the counter medications (OTC) at less cost than a prescription and prescribers should consider his before writing a prescription.

📖 Over the counter drugs (OTCs).

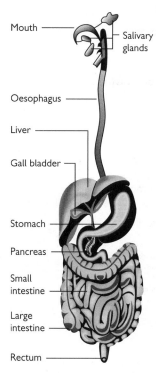

Fig. 12.4 Brief anatomy and physiology of the GI tract. Reproduced from Glasper, EA, McEwing, G, Richardson, J. *Oxford Handbook of Children's and Young People's Nursing*, by kind permission of Oxford University Press.

Oral cavity

The oral cavity comprises:
- cheeks
- lips
- tongue.

Function of the oral cavity
- Speech
- Ingestion
- Chewing (mastication)
- Taste
- Lubrication
- Digestion of starch
- Swallowing (deglutition)
- Respiration.

Xerostomia (dry mouth)
Can result from:
- medication:
  - antiparkinsonian drugs
  - antihistamines
  - lithium
  - monoamine oxidase inhibitors
  - tricyclic antidepressants
  - clonidine
- antimuscarinic drugs
- dehydration
- emotional stress
- radiotherapy
- renal failure
- shock.

Table 12.7 Oral assessment

Area	Normal appearance	Problems
Lips	Smooth	Bleeding
	Pink	Ulceration
	Moist	Cracks at the edges of the mouth
Buccal mucosa	Pink	Reddening
	Moist	Coated (oral candidiasis)
		Ulcerated
Saliva	Clear	Dryness (xerostomia)
Tongue	Pink	Reddening
	Moist	Coated (candidiasis)
	Papillae present	Papillary loss
		Blisters
		Ulceration
		Cracking
Gums	Pink	Bleeding
	Firm	Bleeding with pressure
		Reddened (gingivitis)
		Puffy and pale (oedema)
Teeth	White	Broken teeth
	No evidence of dental caries	Teeth with rough edges
		Plaque
		Dental abscess
Dentures	Well fitting	Rubbing
	Clean	Uneven
		Broken

Oral candidiasis

Those most at risk have altered or compromised autoimmune responses
- debilitated infants and children
- the elderly
- people with diabetes
- those with an indwelling venous or urinary catheter
- those receiving corticosteroid therapy
- those receiving or having recently completed antibiotic therapy
- those with immunodeficiency, e.g. HIV, AIDS, chemotherapy for cancer treatment.

Preparations for the treatment of oral candidiasis

Fluconazole capsules and oral solution
- Contraindications:
  - hepatic impairment
  - previous hypersensitivity
  - increases the effect of warfarin, sulphonylureas, and antiepileptics
  - use with caution in pregnancy.
- Adverse effects
  - nausea
  - abdominal discomfort
  - flatulence
  - diarrhoea
  - impaired liver function
  - angioedema
  - anaphylaxis.

Miconazole oral gel and dental lacquer
- Contraindications:
  - hepatic impairment
  - previous hypersensitivity
  - use with caution in pregnancy.
- Interactions:
  - increases the prothrombin time when administered with warfarin
  - increases blood levels of phenytoin
  - prolongs the serum half-life of sulphonylureas
  - potentiates antiepileptics
  - antagonizes the effect of amphotericin.
- Adverse effects:
  - oral preparation may cause GI upset if used over a long time, i.e. nausea, vomiting, or diarrhoea.
  - headache and rash.

Nystatin pastilles and oral suspension
- Contraindications: previous hypersensitivity.
- Adverse effects: oral irritation; large doses may cause nausea, diarrhoea, vomiting.

The pharynx and oesophagus

This hollow muscular tube links the mouth and stomach.

Heartburn

This region may be affected by heartburn—a retrosternal or epigastric burning sensation which spreads upwards into the pharynx and may spread across the chest.

Mild to moderate heartburn may be helped by:
- lifestyle changes:
  - weight loss
  - smoking cessation
  - reduction in alcohol consumption
  - avoiding large meals especially late at night,
  - raising the head of the bed
  - avoiding foods known to precipitate the condition.
- antacids and alginate–antacids which can be purchased by the patient as an OTC medication.
- If there is minimal or no response to these, an H2-receptor antagonist, which reduces the volume and reduces gastric acid secretion, or a proton pump inhibitor (PPI) may be prescribed.

Note In the young it may be best to try a PPI first as these are more effective.

Table 12.8 Contraindications and adverse effects of H_2-receptor antagonists

Contraindication	Adverse effects
Hepatic impairment	Diarrhoea
Renal impairment	Impaired liver function
Pregnancy	Headache
Breast feeding	Rash
Cimetidine inhibits the action of:	Dizziness
• warfarin	Tiredness
• phenytoin	Rare effects include:
• aminophylline	• bradycardia
• theophylline	• acute pancreatitis
	• confusion
	• depression
	• atrio-ventricular block
	• impotence
	• older people may be affected by hallucinations

Small intestine

It is referred to as 'small' as the lumen has a diameter of only 2.5cm, although it measures 2.0m in length. Composed of three regions:
- the duodenum (approx. 25cm long)
- jejunum (approx. 2.5m)
- ileum (approx. 3.5m).

Gastroenteritis

Caused by infection of the GI tract. Symptoms include:
- abdominal pain
- diarrhoea
- vomiting
- abdominal cramps
- bloating
- flatulence
- nausea
- fever
- faecal urgency
- tenesmus.

Both the young and frail older people are at risk of becoming dehydrated and salt depleted. Dehydration in infants is a medical emergency and referral will be indicated if symptoms do not abate within 24 hrs.

Presenting symptoms of dehydration and salt depletion may be:
- lassitude
- anorexia
- light-headedness
- postural hypotension
- nausea.

Assessment
- Obtain a full history.
- Assess state of hydration.
- Assess frequency and consistency of bowel motions.
- If more than one person is affected, or if symptoms have persisted for more than 4 days, a referral may be indicated.
- If patients have a fever, abdominal pain, blood in the diarrhoea, tenesmus, severe dehydration, shock, or vomiting to the extent they are unable to retain oral rehydration solutions (ORS), referral is indicated.

Preparations for the treatment of gastroenteritis
Rehydration

Give advice and proprietary ORS, such as Dioralyte®, Electrolade®, or Rehidrat®. Once rehydrated, further prevention of dehydration should be avoided by encouraging normal fluid intake and use of ORS to replace additional losses due to vomiting and diarrhoea. Infants should be offered breast or formula feeds in addition to ORS drinks.

Antimotility agents

Useful in non-infectious diarrhoea. Bowel motility is decreased as these narcotic analgesics act upon the opioid μ-receptors on the mesenteric neurons in the intestinal wall, causing a reduction in the release of acetylcholine (📖 Pain), resulting in suppression of peristaltic action.

All antimotility agents

- Contraindications:
  - not to be used for diarrhoea caused by infection because diarrhoea enables invading pathogens to be eliminated.
  - not shown to be useful for children and infants.
- Adverse effects:
  - associated with CNS toxicity and paralytic ileus in the young.

Codeine phosphate

- Contraindications:
  - acute diarrhoeal conditions e.g. ulcerative colitis
  - hypersensitivity to opioids
  - respiratory depression
  - severe respiratory disease
  - acute alcoholism
  - risk of paralytic ileus.
- Adverse effects:
  - drowsiness
  - sedation
  - dizziness
  - lethargy
  - mood changes
  - agitation
  - dependency
  - hallucinations
  - bradycardia
  - palpitations
  - tachycardia
  - hypotension
  - nausea
  - constipation
  - urinary retention
  - flushing
  - rash
  - hypothermia
  - respiratory depression.

Loperamide

A synthetic opioid that does not readily cross the brain–blood barrier.
- Contraindications:
  - those with ulcerative colitis or abdominal distension, where peristaltic inhibition should be avoided.
- Adverse effects:
  - abdominal cramps
  - drowsiness
  - dizziness
  - skin reactions
  - abdominal bloating
  - paralytic ileus.

Antibiotics

Antibiotics are indicated if infection is shown to be caused by:

- *Salmonella*
- *Shigella*
- *Campylobacter*
- *Clostridia*.

Advice should be sought from Public Health on likely pathogens.

Bowel colic

This abdominal pain is caused by spasmodic contractions of the intestine. It may be treated by administration of an antimuscarinic (formerly known as anticholinergic) drug, which both decreases gastrointestinal secretions and acts as a smooth muscle relaxant.

Table 12.9 Cautions, contraindications, and adverse effects of antimuscarinic preparations

Caution	Contraindication	Adverse effects
Antimuscarinic drugs are not be used for people with Down syndrome, children, and older people		These are increased in this group
Caution with their use for people with:	Angle- closure glaucoma	Constipation
• gastro-oesophageal reflux disease	Myasthenia gravis	Transient bradycardia (followed by tachycardia, palpitations, and cardiac arythmias)
• diarrhoea	Paralytic ileus	
• ulcerative colitis	Pyloric stenosis	Reduced bronchial secretions
• acute MI	Prostatic enlargement	
• tachycardia		
• hyperthyroidism		
• cardiac insufficiency following cardiac surgery		Urinary retention and urgency
• pyrexia		Pupil dilation with loss of accommodation
• pregnancy		
• breast feeding		Photophobia
• those receiving antiparkinsonian treatments		
		Dry mouth and skin
		Flushing
For interactions see BNF		Confusion sometimes occurs in the older person

Helminths

Helminths (multicellular parasitic worms), both *Enterobius vermicularis* (thread- or pinworms) and, more rarely, *Ascaris lumbricoides* (roundworms), are found within the digestive tract.

They may be classified as nematodes (roundworms), cestodes (tapeworms), and trematodes (flat worms and flukes).

It is estimated that about 40% of UK schoolchildren under 10 years old have an infestation of threadworms. Transmission rates are particularly high for children living in dense populations with poor sanitary conditions.

Roundworm infestations have a much lower incidence and more serious consequences as they may cause intestinal obstruction or pulmonary eosinophilia. It is most likely that they will have been contracted abroad.

Threadworms

Clinical features

- Nocturnal pruritus
- Worms (8–12 mm long) visible on the perianal skin or in the stools
- Vulvo-vaginitis
- Vaginal discharge.

Treatment

Antihelmetic preparations are available which either prevent the uptake of glucose by the worm (mebendazole), which becomes depleted of energy and dies, or which cause paralysis to the worm by blocking the neurotransmitter acetylcholine (piperazine). The paralysed worm is then removed from the intestine by normal peristaltic activity of the host. A third type of antihelmetic (Pripsen®—piperazine and sennoside) kills the paralysed worm which is expelled along with the faeces.

Re-infestation is common, so two doses of mebendazole may be required, the second dose 2–3 weeks after the first.

The second course of piperazine is usually given for 7 days, 14 days after the first course.

Advice to avoid reinfestation includes:

- treat the whole family if possible.
- cut fingernails short.
- hand washing and scrubbing after using the toilet and before preparing and eating.
- bath or shower on rising to wash away any eggs that have been laid during the night.
- pants or pyjamas to be worn at night and washed daily.
- mittens or gloves may be worn to avoid scratching and carrying the eggs to the mouth. These also need daily laundering.

Preparations for the treatment of helminth infection

Mebendazole
- Contraindications:
  - pregnancy; teratogenesis has been shown in rats
  - not for those under 2 years old, because there is insufficient information regarding safety in these patients.
- Adverse effects:
  - can cross the placenta
  - rare occurrence of abdominal pain or diarrhoea.

Piperazine
- Contraindications:
  - avoid in the first trimester of pregnancy
  - lactating women should not breast feed within 8 hrs of taking
  - avoid in those with: liver disease, renal disease, epilepsy (piperazine lowers the seizure threshold).
- Adverse effects
  - nausea
  - blurred vision
  - vomiting
  - bronchospasm
  - diarrhoea
  - rash
  - adominal cramps
  - anorexia
  - rarely, causes drowsiness, lack of muscle coordination, convulsions.

Large intestine

Consists of:
- caecum: a blind-ended pouch with the appendix projecting. Receives chyme from the ileum via the ileo-caecal valve.
- ascending colon: sodium is reabsorbed along with chloride and water
- transverse colon: sodium is reabsorbed along with chloride and water
- descending colon
- rectum.

Haustral contractions move the contents back and forth along the large intestine, aiding absorption and storing material until the colonic contents are moved into the rectum. Stimulation of the stretch receptors in the rectal wall initiate the defecation reflex (the call to stool).

Constipation (difficulty in passing stools)

Stools of poor bulk, sometimes caused by a diet low in fibre, or hardness, due to increased time in the intestine, or poor hydration may be difficult to pass.

Assessment

Assessment of constipation requires:
- A full history:
  - What is the normal pattern for the individual?
  - Are the changes in bowel habit recent?
  - Family history of bowel cancer?
  - Medical history: is there anything which might predispose to constipation?
  - Drug action, e.g. opiates, aluminium antacids, and anticholinergics can cause constipation.
  - What other symptoms does the patient have?
  - Is fluid intake sufficient?
- Abdominal examination revealing the following indicates an acute condition:
  - a tender abdomen with guarding and rigidity
  - rebound tenderness
  - if the pain is radiating, shifting (where is it, what relieves it?)
  - absent bowel sounds.
- Rectal examination revealing:
  - a full rectum, suggests nerve damage or failure to heed the 'call to stool'
  - an empty rectum, suggests a chronic obstruction or laxative abuse.

NB: only undertake abdominal and rectal examinations if competent to do so.

Treatment

Constipation can be treated with lifestyle changes, such as an increase of foods with dietary fibre (18–30g/day) and an increase in fluid intake (1.5–2 litres) where this has been low. It is important to encourage a response to the 'call to stool', usually shortly after mealtimes, as ignoring this will allow more fluid to be absorbed from the stool, making stools difficult to pass. If there is a poor response to these interventions then laxatives and rectal preparations may be needed.

Laxatives and rectal preparations

Laxatives are medicines that promote bowel evacuation, and may be mild (aperients) or strong (purgative or cathartic). Rectal preparations are either suppositories or enemas.

Bulk forming laxatives

For those with a low fluid, low fibre diet, these laxatives increase the volume of faecal matter, stimulating peristalsis. Some trap water by forming a viscous gel, softening faeces and decreasing transit time. They are useful for those with colostomy or ileostomy.

- Generic names:
  - bran
  - ispaghula (husk granules and powder)
  - sterculia
  - granules
  - methylcellulose.
- Contraindications:
  - difficulty in swallowing
  - intestinal obstruction
  - atonic colon
  - faecal impaction.
- Adverse effects
  - flatulence
  - abdominal distention.

Table 12.10 Possible explanations for symptoms accompanying constipation

Symptom	Possible reason
Increased bowel sounds, abdominal distension, and/or pain	Structural lesion
Thin, pencil-shaped stools	Lesion in the descending colon
Abdominal mass, jaundice, weight loss and fatigue	Advanced colon cancer
Black or malaena stool	High intestinal lesion
Blood mixed with stool	Colonic bleeding
Stool covered with blood	Lower colonic or rectal disease
Blood on toilet paper	Anal fissure, haemorrhoids

Osmotics

Lactulose
- Mode of action: osmotic laxative.
- Semi-synthetic disaccharide, not absorbed from the bowel.
- Contraindications:
  - intestinal obstruction
  - galactosaemia.
- Adverse effects:
  - abdominal cramps
  - flatulence.

Macrogols
- Mode of action:
  - retain water in the large intestine
  - undergo fermentation in the colon, producing gas and short-chain fatty acids stimulating peristalsis
  - discourage the formation of ammonia producing organisms.
- Contraindications:
  - intestinal obstruction
  - paralytic ileus
  - Crohn's disease
  - ulcerative colitis
  - toxic megacolon.
- Adverse effects:
  - abdominal distension
  - nausea
  - abdominal pain.

Magnesium hydroxide, phosphate enema, sodium citrate enema
Contraindications: colic, bowel irritation

Stimulants
Oral and rectal preparations for those on prolonged bed rest with neurological dysfunction, or to counteract other constipating drug therapies. Induce peristaltic action by stimulation of the nerve plexuses to produce propulsive waves.

Senna, dantron, sodium picosulfate
- Contraindications:
  - avoid in intestinal obstruction
  - avoid with children
  - use with caution in pregnancy.
- Adverse effects:
  - gripe
  - abdominal cramps.

Bisacodyl

- Contraindications:
  - avoid in intestinal obstruction
  - avoid with children
  - use with caution in pregnancy.
- Adverse effects:
  - gripe
  - abdominal cramps
  - may cause rectal irritation.

Glycerol suppositories

Docusate (tablets, oral solution, or enema): docusate sodium reduces the surface tension of stools, allowing fluid to enter and soften, in addition to stimulation of peristalsis.

- Contraindications:
  - do not use oral formula in intestinal obstruction or for those with nausea, vomiting, or abdominal pain
  - avoid rectal preparations if rectal fissures or haemorrhoids.
- Adverse effects of oral formulation:
  - cramps
  - nausea
  - anorexia.
- Liquid paraffin is no longer used due to:
  - impaired fat-soluble vitamin absorption
  - potential inhalation of droplets causing lipid pneumonia
  - anal seepage of oil
  - prolonged use has a risk of cancer.

Faecal lubricants/softeners

Soften faeces and lubricate bowel to promote motility. Softeners are used for patients who need to avoid straining, e.g. after surgery, MI.

Arachis oil

Use warmed to soften impacted faeces.

Table 12.11 When and how to take laxative preparations

Type of product	When to take	Specifics
Bulk formers	Do not take before bed	Should be taken with water and consumed as soon as the fibres swell
Osmotics	Lactulose: take with water or fruit juice	Lactulose: may take 48 hrs to work
	Magnesium hydroxide: shake well before taking and take with water	Magnesium hydroxide: 2–4 hrs before effect
		Macrogols: avoid in pregnancy and breast feeding. discontinue if fluid or electrolyte imbalance
Stimulants	Senna: take with fluid	Senna: make take 8–12 hrs to work
	Bisacodyl: take after food and 1 hr after or before other medications	Bisacodyl: taken orally, effect in 10–12 hrs; suppository, 20–60 mins
	Dantron: take at bedtime	Dantron: effect in 6–12 hrs. Incontinent patients: avoid prolonged contact with skin (risk of irritation/ excoriation). Avoid in pregnancy and breast feeding
		Glycerin suppositories- moisten with water and insert into faeces
Stimulant/softeners/lubricants	Oral docusate sodium: take alone or 1 hr after or before other medications	Oral docusate: take with water, effect in 1–2 days
		Arachis enema: warm to body heat. Needs to be retained for as long as possible for maximum effect

Prescribing for the prevention and treatment of infections

Immune response

Specific immunity

Provided by the lymphocytes, both T and B cells act as a coordinated response to specific antigens. T cells are responsible for the mediation of cell immunity providing defense against abnormal cells and pathogens inside cells. B cells respond to antigens and pathogens in body fluids providing humeral or antibody-mediated immunity.

Vaccines

Vaccines provoke a response to a particular pathogen, which is intentionally administered in order to sensitise the immune cells for a subsequent exposure and protect the individual. Immunoglobulin refers to antibodies of a human origin. Antiserum refers to materials prepared in animals.

Adverse effects

These vary from a few symptoms to a mild form of the disease, including fever and malaise and discomfort at the site of the injection.

Post-immunisation Pyrexia – Joint committee on Vaccination and Immunisation recommendation

Parents should be informed if pyrexia develops following childhood immunization and the child should be given a dose of paracetamol, suitable to their age and weight. This may be followed by a second dose 6–8 hours later if symptoms persist (see Table 12.13). Medical advice should be sought if pyrexia persists after the second dose.
See literature accompanying the product for full details of side effects and contra-indications.

Anaphylactic reactions These are rare but serious as they may prove fatal.

Table 12.11 Forms of immunity

Type of immunity	How acquired
Innate immunity	Present at birth Genetically determined No relationship to exposure to antigens
Acquired immunity	Not present at birth Either active or passive
Active acquired immunity	Naturally acquired immunity following exposure to an antigen within the environment or induced active immunity following deliberate exposure to an antigen i.e. vaccination or immunization
Passive acquired immunity	Natural passive immunity following the transfer of antibodies from another person i.e a mother to her baby either in utero via the placenta or in breast milk, or induced passive immunity when antibodies are administered in the form of antisera to prevent or fight infection

Table 12.12 Types of vaccine

Type of vaccine	Characteristic	Number of doses
Inactivated preparations	The organism is treated with heat or chemically in order to render it safe Stimulates antibody response but not cell mediated immunity	May require a series of administrations initially followed by boosters
Attenuated organisms e.g. Poliomyelitis	Viable organisms which cause infection but not disease Stimulation both cell mediated and humoral immunity	Immunization generally achieved by a single dose
Extracts of detoxified exotoxins	In some organisms the disease is caused by a reaction to the toxins The vaccination is by a chemically treated toxin so toxicity is lost but antigenicity remains	Requires a series of administrations initially followed by boosters

Table 12.13 Doses of paracetamol for post immunization pyrexia in children

Age	Dose by mouth	Comments
2 months	60 mg (10mg/kg if jaundiced)	For post immunization pyrexia only, otherwise do not give to a baby under 3 months of age
3 months–1 year	60–120 mg	
1–5 years	120–250 mg	
6–12 years	250–500 mg	

Prescribing tips

- Vaccines which are available for nurse prescribers who are trained and competent in their administration, contraindications and the recognition and management of anaphylaxis are listed in the CPF.
- In general, if the patient is suffering an acute illness postpone vaccination.
- A severe reaction to a preceding dose is a contraindication for further doses and boosters.
- Hypersensitivity to hen's eggs contraindicates influenza vaccine.
- Live vaccines should not be routinely administered to pregnant women, individuals with impaired immune response or those with leukaemia
  Avoid the intra muscular route for patients with bleeding disorders

NB: doses may be repeated every 4–6 hrs when necessary, do not exceed more than 4 doses in any 24 hour period.

Oral syringes may be obtained from the pharmacy to ensure the correct dose/volume is given.

Treatment of bacterial infections

Know your bacteria

The cell walls of bacteria contain a unique substance called peptidoglycan. Penicillins, penicillinase-resistant penicillins and cephalosporins disrupt the formation of the peptidoglycan layer of the cell wall, thus inhibiting the maintenance of the cells osmotic gradient resulting in the cell rupturing and dying.

Polymixins bind to phospholipids within the cell membrane altering its permeability and allowing holes to form within the membrane resulting in the cell rupturing.

Bacterial cells differ in other ways from those of the human body:

- The permeable cell membrane contains no sterols.
- The cell lacks a nucleus. Genetic material, DNA, is found within a single chromosome lying in the cell cytoplasm.
- Quinolones disrupt the replication of cell DNA especially blocking the activity of DNA gyrase essential for DNA replication and repair.
- Similarly, metronidazole breaks down and inhibits synthesis of bacterial DNA.
- Both preparations which stimulate the immune system providing protection from an assault and those which treat an established infection are available in the CPF.

Choice of a suitable drug

There are two main considerations:

The patient

- Their history of allergy.
- Hepatic and renal function.
- Are they immunocompromised?
- Ability to tolerate oral medication.
- If female whether pregnant, breast feeding, or taking the oral contraceptive.
- Their ethnic origins.
- Their age.

The likely causative organism

- Its sensitivity.
- Safety for particular patient group.
- Local antibacterial policies.
- Is it a notifiable disease?
- Duration of treatment.
- Dosage according to age, weight, renal function, severity of the infection.
- Route of administration.
- Contra-indications.

Remember

- Viral infections should not be treated with antibacterials.
- Antibacterials should not be prescribed prophylactically.
- Specific timings of some antibacterials.

Table 12.14 Antibacterial drugs

Classification	Mode of action	Mechanism	Examples
Bacteriostatic	Inhibit bacterial growth without killing the cell	Modification of bacterial energy metabolism	Tremethoprim
	The human immune system will eventually destroy the bacteria	Protein synthesis inhibitors	Tetracyclines
Bactericidal	Kill the bacteria	Inhibition of synthesis and damage to the cell wall or membrane	Penicillin
By chemical structure	Quinolones (synthetic anti-microbial agents) inhibit replication of bacterial DNA and prevent the bacteria form replication and repair.	Modification of bacterial nucleic acid or protein synthesis	Ciprofloxacin
	Others bind to the subunits of the bacterial ribosomes where proteins are synthesized.		

Table 12.15 Optimal administration times and methods

Preparation	Timing	Reason
Tetracycline	1 hour before meals or 2 hours after	Absorption is adversely affected by dairy products
	Should be swallowed whole, whilst sitting or standing	
Nitrofurantoin	After meals	To avoid gastric irritation

Prescribing for pain

The physiology of pain

Sensations of pain are transmitted from nociceptors to the central nervous system (CNS). Nociceptors are found in the epidermal layer of the skin, joint capsules, periostea of bone, and in the walls of blood vessels. Nociceptors have a large receptive field and this makes it difficult to pin point the exact source of a painful sensation. Pain may be perceived as sharp and localized, diffuse, or referred.

Nociceptors may be sensitive to:
- Extremes of temperature
- Mechanical damage
- Chemicals such as those which signal damaged cells.

Strong stimuli may excite all of these receptors.

During injury, tissue damage occurs to the cell membrane which releases arachidonic acid into the interstitial fluid in the injured area. This is converted by the enzyme cyclo-oxygenase into different types of pro staglandins. Prostaglandins co-ordinate cellular activity and stimulate nociceptors in the area surrounding the injury.

Thus the initial reaction to an injury is sharp localized pain followed by a more diffuse discomfort.

The action of aspirin (acetylsalicylic acid) and other NSAIDs

Aspirin and other NSAIDs act by:
- Reversibly (most NSAIDs) or irreversibly (aspirin) inactivating cyclo-oxygenase, which suppresses the production of prostaglandins in response to injury.
- action is therefore local rather than centrally involving the brain.
- body's response to pyrexia is the release of prostaglandins in the brain, which causes the hypothalamus to reset the body's thermostat at the new higher level in an attempt to preserve stasis. Aspirin enables the normal body temperature to be restored.

Aspirin is therefore suitable for use with mild to moderate pain such as headache, muscular pain and dysmenorrhea, and in pyrexia. Adult dose is 300–900 mg, every 4–6 hrs, with a maximum of 4g daily.
📖 Basic principles of pharmacology.

Interactions

Table 12.16 Drugs that interact with aspirin

Drug	Effect of aspirin
Anticoagulants	Increased risk of bleeding due to antiplatelet effect
Antacids and adsorbents	Increased urine alkalinity
	Increased excretion of aspirin
Antiepileptics e.g. phenotoin and valporate	Enhances the effect of phenotoin and valporate
Corticosteriods	Increased risk of:
	• gastrointestinal bleeding
	• gastrointestinal ulceration
Cytotoxics	Reduced excretion rate
	Increased toxicity
Diuretics	Antagonism of diuretic effect of spironalactone
	Reduced excretion of acetazolamide (risk of toxicity)
Metoclopramide	Increased rate of aspirin absorption
Mifepristone	Avoid aspirin until 8–12 days after taking mifepristone
Uricosurics	Reduction in effects of probenecid and sulphinpyrazone

Adverse effects of aspirin

Table 12.17 Side effects and contraindications of aspirin

Area	Side effects	Comments
Gastric	Irritates gastric mucosa Can cause nausea and vomiting Gastric ulceration Gastric bleeding Exacerbation of peptic ulceration Erosive gastritis	Inhibits prostaglandin production decreasing production of gastric mucus Can lead to mucosal damage and bleeding (blood loss of 10–30ml per day) To reduce these effects take after food
Anticoagulation	Blood vessels damaged in tissue injury By inhibiting the enzyme cyclo-oxygenase, aspirin inhibits platelet aggregation	Has an anticoagulatory effect In large doses may prolong the bleeding time Should not be prescribed for people with haemophilia
Hypersensitivity	Attacks of asthma, angioedema, urticaria, and rhinitis have been precipitated by aspirin	Caution: 1 in 10 patients with asthma or allergic conditions may be hypersensitive to aspirin
Renal and Hepatic disease	Can cause liver and kidney impairment	Those with these conditions should avoid Aspirin
Pregnancy	If taken in the 3rd trimester it can: • cause fetal abnormalities • prolong pregnancy and labour • cause excessive bleeding before, during and after delivery	Avoid if possible in the last few weeks of pregnancy
Reye's syndrome	Can cause Reye's syndrome in children under 12 years Symptoms involve a combination of: • swelling of the brain • liver inflammation • avoid using aspirin during or • following a viral infection as this may trigger Raye's syndrome in children under 12 years of age.	Do not give aspirin to children under 12 years Do not give to breast feeding mothers
Toxicity	Tinnitus Hearing loss Hyperventilation Respiratory acidosis Fever	Toxicity occurs when daily dosage exceeds 4g

NSAID administration routes

NSAIDs may be administered by several routes.
- Orally.
- Some topically.
- Diclofenac rectally.
- Some by injection, for musculoskeletal pain e.g. acute low back pain. The side effects are the same as for oral administration with the additional problem of painful injections.
- Diclofenac must be given by deep intra muscularly (IM) injection (not IV as this may cause venous thrombosis)—dose 75mg (repeated if necessary after 30 mins max dose in 24hrs—150mg).
- Ketrolac may be given IM or slowly IV (see latest BNF).

Adverse effects of other NSAIDs

As with aspirin these can cause gastrointestinal irritation, bleeding and perforation, with increased risk at higher doses and in those over 60 years of age or with a history of peptic ulcer.
NSAIDs may:
- exacerbate asthma
- precipitate renal failure in those with heart failure, cirrhosis or renal insufficiency.

Contraindications of other NSAIDs

- Use with caution with older people.
- In allergic disorders, asthma, urticaria or rhinitis, and those with a hypersensitivity to aspirin.
- During pregnancy and breast feeding.
- Those with coagulation defects.
- Long term use may cause reduced fertility in women which is reduced on cessation of treatment.

Interaction of other NSAIDs

See latest BNF Appendix 1 NSAIDs interactions.

Many NSAIDs can cause serious side effects but ibuprofen, diclofenac, and naproxen are relatively safe. Ibuprofen has the lowest incidence of side effects, is the cheapest, and may be purchased as an OTC medication.

Ibuprofen is useful as both an analgesic and antipyretic in children when paracetamol is insufficient. See NICE guidelines (🖳 www.nice. org.uk) on cyclo-oxygenase-2 selective inhibitors.

Table 12.18 NSAID dosage

Name	Timing	Adult doses	Child doses
Ibuprofen	3–4 divided doses	1.2–1.8g daily PO (max. 2.4g daily)	(>7 kg) 20 mg/kg in 3–4 divided doses
Diclofenac (oral or rectal)	2–3 divided doses	75–150mg daily PO	–
Naproxen	2 divided doses	0.5–1g daily PO (max. 1.25g daily)	–

Paracetamol

Similar analgesic and antipyretic properties to aspirin but is not an anti-inflammatory agent. It is thought to work by inhibiting the production of cyclo-oxygenase in the CNS and to have an effect on peripheral pain receptors.

It is suitable for mild to moderate pain.

Adverse effects

Paracetamol has relatively few adverse effects compared with aspirin however the toxic level is little greater than the therapeutic level and overdosage is particularly dangerous as it may cause liver damage which is sometimes not apparent for 4–6 days.

In overdose, the liver is unable to provide sufficient amounts of the protein glutathione which counteracts the highly toxic metabolite, acetyl-benzo-quinoneimine, formed during the breakdown of paracetamol in the liver.

There is a possibility of accidental overdose as many OTC medications for pain, sinus problems, or cold and flu symptom relief contain paracetamol alone or in combination with other drugs. It is vital to ask patients to check the active ingredients in any other remedy they may be taking and not to take more than one paracetamol-containing preparation at a time.

Paracetamol can be used safely for children and pregnant and breast feeding women and is also suitable for use with older people.

Contraindications

There are no contraindications however use is cautioned for those with hepatic or renal impairment or those who suffer from alcohol dependence.

Interactions

See current BNF appendix regarding paracetamol.

Table 12.19 Doses of paracetamol

Age group	Dose (PO)	Timing	Max. dose
Adult	0.5–1 g	4–6 hourly	4g daily
Children: 2 months (post immunisation pyrexia)	60 mg 10mg per kg or if jaundiced*		
3 months –1 year	60–120 mg	4–6 hourly	4 doses in 24 hrs
1–5 years	120–250 mg	4–6 hourly	4 doses in 24 hrs
6–12 years	250–500 mg	4–6 hourly	4 doses in 24 hrs

* See Post-immunisation Pyrexia Joint Committee on Vaccination and Immunisation recommendations

The action of opioid analgesics

Opioids act on receptors in the CNS which are designed for the endogenous opiods and therefore have no anti-inflammatory effects. The opioid receptors suppress pain messages from the periphery to the CNS. Each receptor has been designated a letter of the Greek alphabet, mu (μ), kappa (κ), episilon (ε) and delta (δ).

Adverse effects of opiates

Morphine, codeine, and pethidine all mimic the action of endogenous opiates providing both pain relief and other unwanted effects such as:
- respiratory depression
- constipation
- drowsiness
- hypotension
- bradycardia
- tachycardia
- drowsiness
- sedation
- miosis
- anorexia
- flushing
- urticaria
- nausea
- urinary retention
- hypotension.

Opioids are used for the relief of moderate to severe pain. There is a risk with repeated administration of the patient becoming tolerant or dependent on these drugs. This should not be a deterrent for their use in the management of pain for people with pain in a terminal illness.

Contraindications of opioid analgesics

Codeine phosphate (a morphine salt) is contraindicated in respiratory disease and for those with respiratory depression or a hypersensitivity to opioids.

Interactions

- See appendix in the latest BNF.
- There is a special hazard with pethidine and perhaps other opioids and monoamine oxidase inhibitors (MAOIs).

Table 12.20 Opioid receptors and their corresponding endogenous opioid

Receptor	Position	Endogenous opioid	Action
Mu (μ)	Dorsal horn of the spinal chord and thalamus	Endogenous β-endorphin	Analgesia Respiratory depression Euphoria
Kappa (κ)	Hypothalamus	Dynorphin	Analgesia Sedation Miosis Hypothermia
Epsilon (ε)	Hippocampus and amygdala	Enkephalin	Some psychotic effects Dysphoria
Delta (δ)	Limbic system	Unknown	Behavioral change Hallucinations

Prescribing for neuropathic pain

Neuropathic pain results from damage to neural tissue.
- Post herpetic neuralgia
- Phantom limb pain
- Compression neuropathies
- Peripheral neuropathies
- Pain following stroke
- Spinal chord injury
- Syringomyelia
- Idiopathic neuropathy.

Treatment
- Tricyclic antidepressants are usually used for treatment of neuropathic pain. Some antiepileptic drugs may also be suitable.
- Opioids are only partially effective for this type of pain but may be considered if other treatments fail.
- The use of transcutaneous electrical nerve stimulation (TENS) may help, as may topical application of capsaicin cream.
- Compression neuropathy may be eased by the use of corticosteroid preparations.

Local anaesthetics (LA)

Local anaesthetics may be applied to the mucous membrane or injected. They cause a reversible block to the transmission of pain signals along the nerve pathway. The variation of preparation determines its applicability to the route of administration, which may be:

- topical
- epidural
- local infiltration
- nerve blocks.

Administration

It is important to consider the rate at which the preparations are absorbed and excreted and the potency of the product. Considerations include:

- the duration of the procedure
- a person's:
  - weight
  - age
  - clinical condition
- vascularity in the area to be anaesthetized.

Contraindications

- Poor cooperation or refusal by the patient.
- Allergy to local anaesthetic; anaphylaxis is rare but can occur:
  - check specific details of any reported allergy.
  - check if allergic symptoms were a response to overdose, or a faint caused by pain or fear rather than a reaction.
- Infection at the proposed site of injection. Injecting into this area could spread the infection. Inflammation may cause high tissue acidity which ↓ effectiveness of LA drugs
- Bleeding disorders, anticoagulant therapy and thrombocytopenia are contraindications for nerve block procedures.

Side effects

↑ risk of toxicity in:

- small children
- older people or those in poor clinical condition
- people with heart block
- low cardiac output
- epilepsy
- myasthenia gravis
- hepatic impairment
- porphyria
- anti-arrhythmic or β-blocker therapy (↑ risk of myocardial depression)
- cimetidine therapy (inhibits the metabolism of lignocaine/lidocaine).

Prescribing for the respiratory tract

Brief anatomy and physiology of the respiratory tract

The respiratory tract comprises
- upper respiratory tract—nose, nasal cavity, and pharynx
- lower respiratory tract—larynx (voice box), trachea (wind pipe), bronchi, lungs containing bronchioles and alveoli.

Structure of the upper respiratory tract
The nose and nasal cavity
- Two nasal passages.
- Rich blood supply and secretory cells to keep them warm and moist. Produce up to 1L of mucus in 24 hrs.
- Providing warm, moist air to the lungs.
- Lines with nasal hairs and cila to remove dust particles.

The pharynx
- Muscular tube leading from the oral cavity and nose to larynx and oesophagus.
- Containing lymphoid tissue the adenoids (nasopharyngeal tonsils) and palatine and lingual tonsils.
- These lymph glands filter out invading micro-organisms.

Structure of the lower respiratory tract
The larynx
- A cartilaginous box containing the epiglottis, which stops ingested materials from entering the bronchi.
- The vocal chords.

The trachea
- C-shaped cartilage ribs keep this tube open.
- Lining of secretory cells.

The lungs
- Cone shaped.
- Divided into lobes.
- Right lung has 3 lobes, left lung has 2 lobes.

The bronchi
- Divided into the right and left branches.
- Right bronchi to the right lung, left to the left lung.
- C-shaped cartilage ribs keep these tubes open.
- Tree like configuration.
- Each bronchi divides to form narrower passages called bronchioles.

The bronchioles
- Further branches are called terminal bronchioles.
- These divide into finer tubes called respiratory bronchioles.
- Terminating in the alveoli.

The alveoli
- Rich capillary blood supply to facilitate gas exchange.
- Approximately 150 million in each lung.

Drugs for the respiratory system
- Respiratory stimulants
- Pulmonary surfactants
- Oxygen
- Muscolytes
- Aromatic inhalers
- Cough suppressants
- Expectorants and demulcent preparations
- Mouthwashes.

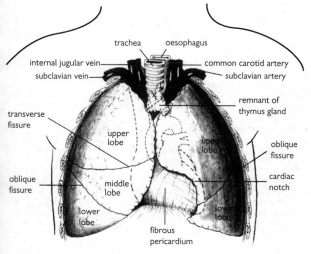

Fig. 12.5 Illustration of the respiratory system

Common conditions

The common cold (coryza)

Definition
- Acute nasopharyngitis

Epidemiology
- Most frequently occurring upper respiratory tract condition
- Very contagious
- Spread by droplets when sneezing and coughing
- Spread by direct contact.

Causes
- Viral
- Local inflammation caused by immunological response
- Micro-organisms are contained in the mucus produced in response to the inflammation.

Signs and symptoms
- Red and swollen nose
- Extra secretion of clear fluid
- Coughing
- Sneezing
- Low grade fever
- Muscular aches.

Treatment
- Pain relief
- Relief of fever
- Topical nasal decongestants
- OTC cold remedies containing decongestant and pain relief combinations.
- Steam inhalations.

Acute sore throat (pharyngitis, laryngitis, or tonsillitis)
Definition
- Tonsillitis—acute inflammation of the tonsils
- Laryngitis—acute inflammation of the larynx
- Pharyngitis—acute inflammation of the pharynx.

Causes
Tonsillitis
- Usually viral
- Bacteria—commonly group A beta haemolytic *streptococcus*.

Laryngitis:
Often in individuals with respiratory infections such as pneumonia or bronchitis.

Pharyngitis:
Oedema of the vocal chords.

Signs and symptoms
Sore throat
- Inflammation of the larynx leading to hoarseness of the voice
- Extra secretion of clear fluid
- Coughing
- Sneezing
- Low grade fever
- Muscular aches.

Treatment
- Pain relief
- Gargling
- Mouthwash
- Treat symptoms
- Increase fluid intake
- If confident bacterial case then antibiotics.

Allergic rhinitis

May be self limiting and not require any treatment.

Definition

Nasal passage has hypersensitive responses to allergens such as pollen.

Causes

- Pollen activates mast cells in the nasal passages.
- Mast cells release histamine and other mediators.
- Histamine acts on receptors in the lining of the nasal passages.
- This causes vasodilation and increased capillary permeability.

Signs and symptoms

- Sneezing
- Watery discharge
- Swollen mucous membranes which lead to narrowing of the airways
- Itchy eyes
- Watering eyes.

Treatment

- Topical nasal corticosteriods.
- Oral and topical antihistamines.
- Systemic nasal decongestants.
- If seasonal condition, begin treatment 2–3 weeks before the triggering pollen is in the environment.

Further reading

Department of Health (2003) *Immunisation against infectious diseases—Pneumococcal.* DoH London.

File T M Jr (2002) New Millennium: new antimicrobial agents for respiratory infections: but an old plea. *Curr. Opin. Infect. Dis* **13** (2).

Low D E (2000) Trends and significance of antimicrobial resistance in respiratory pathogens. *Curr. Opin. Microbiol.* **13** (2).

Public Health Laboratory Service (1997) *Clostridium difficile infection. Prevention and management.* Department of Public health London.

Redding S W (2001) The role of yeasts other than Candida albimcans in oropharangeal candidiasis. *Currr. Opin. Infec. Dis.* **14** (6).

Wood S F (2003) Sneezing, runny, blocked or itchy nose: is it hay fever a cold or something else? *Nurse Prescribing* **1** (2).

Prescribing for skin problems

Brief anatomy and physiology of skin

Structure of the skin

- Largest organ in the human body, surface area of approximately 2m^2
- Limits water loss through this surface area to approx 500 ml each day.
- 16% of an individual's body weight.
- Comprises the outer epidermis and inner dermis.
- Structure varies depending on position in the body, i.e. hairy areas such as the scalp have a thin epidermis, and the non-hairy palms of the hands and soles of the feet have a thicker epidermis.
- Skin structure varies in relation to age, environment, and ethnicity.
- Accessory structures such as, hair, nails, sweat, and sebaceous glands are located within the dermis but protrude through the epidermis.

Epidermis

- Provides protection from mechanical and micro-organism assault
- Outermost layer—stratum corneum.
- Innermost layer—stratum germinativum—is attached to the basement membrane which forms the barrier between epidermis and dermis.
- Stratum germinativum generates new cells to replace those shed at the epithelial surface.
- As cells move towards the surface of the skin their structure and functions change:
  - initially at the basement membrane they begin forming a protein, keratin
  - during their journey to the surface they continue this protein synthesis
  - on reaching the surface some 15–30 days later, their internal organelles have gone and they are flattened capsules of protein
- They remain in the stratum corneum for 14 days, providing a protective barrier:
  - first, this barrier, rich in lipids, limits the loss of water through the skin's surface
  - secondly, the keratin within each flattened cell enables the retention of water molecules.

Dermis

- A network of proteins, collagen and elastin:
  - elastin provides flexibility to the skin
  - collagen provides strength.
- Accessory structures, i.e. sweat glands, are found throughout the dermal area, whereas sebaceous glands are only in hairy areas.

Function of the skin

- Protection of underlying structures.
- Maintenance of body temperature.
- Storage of nutrients.
- Excretion of waste, i.e. salt, water.
- Sensory detection of temperature, pain, etc.
- Protection from mechanical and micro-organism assault.

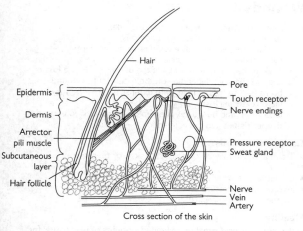

Cross section of the skin

Fig. 12.6 Brief anatomy and physiology of the skin. Reproduced from Glasper, EA, McEwing, G, Richardson, J. *Oxford Handbook of Children's and Young People's Nursing*, by kind permission of Oxford University Press.

Wounds

- Wounds are classified depending on their depth:
  - superficial wounds affect the epidermis
  - partial thickness wounds extend as far as the dermis
  - full thickness wounds involve fat or deeper layers.
- A break in the external integrity of the dermis leads to a loss of function of the skin, depending on the nature of the wound:
  - burns lead to loss of fluid, with extensive burns this may be a life-threatening loss
  - lacerations and punctures allow micro-organisms to enter the deeper tissues and cause infection.

Causes of wounds

- Trauma, which may be chemical, physical, or mechanical
- Surgery
- Ischaemia (e.g. arterial leg ulcers)
- Pressure (e.g. pressure sores, corns, foot ulcers)
- Or the above in combination.

Healing

- *Primary intention*: formation of limited amounts of new tissue; for example, wounds closed by sutures.
- Wounds caused by trauma may involve new tissue to fill the gap and a covering of epithelium; this is *secondary intention* healing.
- The healing processes of both primary and secondary intention have three overlapping phases:
  - inflammation: red, hot, swollen, and painful
  - proliferation
  - maturation.

Inflammation

- Initial bleeding at the wound site brings fibrinogen, which brings the edges into close approximation, and fibrin, which forms the blood clot.
- The blood clot dries to a scab, preventing bacterial invasion and further fluid loss.
- Serum proteins and white cells leak from adjacent blood vessels.
- This gives rise to the appearance of inflammation (see above).
- Neutrophils and macrophages move into the area to clear any debris and bacteria.

Proliferation

- New blood vessels are formed in a collagen matrix (granulation).
- Wound contracts.
- Epithelialization: epithelial cells on the wounds surface grow down under the dried scab.

Maturation

- Numbers of blood vessels decrease.
- Collagen and scar tissue gradually reshape to normal tissue.

Assessment

History

- General health
- Social circumstances
- Environment.

Routine physical examination

- Position, size, and depth of the wound.
- Is the tissue sloughy-covered or filled with soft yellow slough?
- Necrotic—covered with a hard black layer.
- How much exudate?
- Any signs of infection?
- Presence or absence of pain?
- Clean with significant tissue loss (granulating).
- Clean and superficial (epithelializing).

Wound dressings

Functions

- Maintenance of high humidity (speeds up epithelial growth, reduces pain, and breaks down necrotic tissue).
- Dries excess exudates, preventing tissue maceration.
- Allows gaseous exchange; thought to be beneficial.
- Thermal insulation: a temp of 37°C promotes macrophage and mitotic activity during granulation and formation of epithelial tissue.
- Impermeability to bacteria by reduction of contact with the air.
- Freedom from contaminates and particles.
- Ability to replace without causing trauma to the healing wound.

Assessment

- Essential to fit the type of dressing to the needs of the wound (see below).
- See physical examination above.

📖 History taking.
📖 Clinical and physical examination.

Further reading

Dealey C (1994). *The care of wounds*. Blackwell Science, Oxford.
Dunford C (1997). Management of recurrent pilonidal sinus. *Nursing Times*, **93**(32), 64.
National Prescribing Centre advice about head lice. 🖥 www.npc.co.uk/nurse_prescribing/pdfs/factsOflice.pdf

Terms used to describe injuries to the skin

Table 12.21 Terms used to describe injuries to the skin

Term	Definition	Treatment
Abrasions	A scraping injury which produces a break in the epithelium	Clean Cover or leave open depending on severity
Acne	Disease of the sebaceous glands	Antimicrobials Retinoids Keratolytics
Animal or human bite	Abrasion, laceration, or puncture wound caused by an animal or human bite	As for abrasion Consider tetanus cover Consider antibiotic cover
Atopic dermatitis or eczema	Inflammatory skin disorder	Emollients Creams Ointments
Boils; carbuncles, folliculitis, furuncles	Bacterial infection of the hair follicles which may spread to deeper tissues	Generally resolve without treatment Consider pain relief If spreading consider antibiotics
Burns:	Tissue damage or loss caused by exposure to:	As for abrasion Consider pain relief Consider tetanus cover
thermal	flame, steam, or hot liquid	
chemical	acid or a base	
electrical	electrical current	
radiation	sunburn or radiation treatment	
Candidiasis	Infection of the skin usually caused by Candida albicans	Imidazoles Corticosteriods Topical antifungals Clean the skin
Chronic skin ulcer Caused by:	Blistered, broken, or necrotic skin lesions which may extend to underlying structures	Metronidazole Silver sulfadiazine
1. Pressure sores (decubitus ulcer)	Impaired mobility causing long-term pressure on bony prominences	Move the patient frequently
2. Leg ulcers	Loss of skin to the leg or foot which takes more than 6 weeks to heal	Use appropriate mattress aids, etc.
3. Foot ulcers		If ankle brachial pressure index (ABPI) is <0.8 multilayer compression bandaging is indicated

Table 12.21 (contd.)

Term	Definition	Treatment
Dermatitis		Identify and avoid cause where possible
1. Contact	Localized inflammatory reaction caused by chemical irritant, hypersensitivity, or an allergen	Emollients Topical corticosteroids
2. Seborrhoeic (cradle cap in infants)	Inflammatory disorder involving the scalp, eyebrows, eyelids, ear canals, nasolabial folds, axillae and trunk	Topical antifungals Corticosteroid gels and lotions Betamethasone 0.05% ointment Betamethasone 0.05% in alcoholic-based scalp preparation Desoximetasone 0.25% and salicylic acid 1% lotion Lithium succinate 8% and zinc sulphate 0.05% ointment Ketoconazole 2% shampoo
Dermatophytosis (ringworm)	Fungal infection of the stratum corneum of the skin, the nails and the hair	Topical application of: Imidazoles Clotrimazole
Tinea corporis	Annular lesion with a raised scaly edge with the centre clear	
Tinea cruris (rare in women common in young males)	Scaly erythematous rash of the inner aspects of both thighs and sometimes the buttocks	Terbinafine cream
Tinea pedis (athlete's foot)	Itchy, flaky area of skin; often between the fourth and fifth toes	Miconazole Sulconazole
Tinea versicolour	Rash of the head and neck affecting all age groups	
Herpes labialis	Lesion found on the face and mouth caused by the herpes simplex virus	Usually self-limiting Aciclovir 5% cream Penciclovir 1% cream Consider analgesia
Impetigo	*Staph. aureus* vesicular infection with a honey-coloured discharge which dries to a crust	Tetracycline hydrochloride 3% ointment Flucloxacillin capsules

Table 12.21 (contd.)

Term	Definition	Treatment
Nappy rash	Rash caused by degradation of urine to release ammonia often accompanied by bacterial or fungal infections	Frequent nappy changing Barrier creams Topical mild corticosteroids with antifungals if necessary
Pediculosis (lice infestation)	Infestation of Anoplura or sucking parasites of humans	Malathion Carbaryl
Pediculus humanus capitis (head lice)	Itchy scalp with lesions which may become infected caused by scratching	Pyrethroids In addition: head lice may be treated by mechanical clearance using a fine-toothed comb
Pediculus corporis (body lice)	A red itchy rash with excoriated skin and a pigmented eczema	For body lice, wash clothes and bedding
Pthirus pubis (pubic lice)	Itching is the main symptom	
Sarcoptes scabiei (scabies)	Infestation by the female mite which burrows into the stratum corneum and lays its eggs at the boundary of the dermis and epidermis	Malathion Alcoholic lotion or aqueous lotion Permethrin dermal cream
	Itching is an allergic reaction to the mite's coat, saliva and faeces	Treat the entire household Launder clothing and bedding
	Areas which have been scratched may become infected	
Urticaria (hives or nettle rash)	Allergic skin reaction causing oedema with surrounding erythema and itching	Oral histamines

For more information go to ⌨ www.nurse_prescriber.co.uk or
⌨ www.npc.co.uk/nurse_prescribing

Types of dressing

Alginates

- Contain calcium alginate, a derivative of seaweed.
- Exudate from the wound causes a change in structure in the dressing from fibrous to a gel.
- Different forms: flat dressings, rope or ribbon, or extra-absorbent with an adhesive backing.
- Depending on the product used, the resultant gel can be lifted off as a sheet or it may it require rinsing off.
- Require a secondary dressing to preserve moisture.
- Used for wounds with a heavy exudates and odour.
- May be left in place for up to 7 days. If heavy exudates or infection, dressing may require changing daily.

Contraindications

- Not for infected wounds.
- Unsuitable for dry, necrotic wounds.
- Not to be used with topical antimicrobial or antibiotic agents as these may prevent the gelling process.

Problems

Certain alginates will cause excoriation and maceration of the surrounding skin. (If using Kaltostat® the dressing should be cut and folded to fit the wound.)

Foam dressings

- Promote healing by absorbing exudates and maintaining a moist environment.
- Different preparations are available for wounds which are lightly exudating and for wounds with a heavy exudate.
- Require a secondary dressing.
- *Lyofoam*®
  - Suitable for smelly, moderately exudating wounds.
  - Has an adhesive waterproof backing.
  - Need to overlap the wound by 2–3 cm.
  - Initially change each day, but as discharge deceases can leave for up to 7 days.
- *Allevyn*®
  - Plastic net covered polyurethane foam, bonded to a vapour-permeable polyurethane film backing.
  - The backing is water and bacteria proof.
  - Can be left on a clean, non-infected wound for 3–4 days.
- *Syprosorb*®
  - Layered absorbent polyurethane foam vapour-permeable dressing.
  - Used for wounds with light to moderate exudate.
  - Change dressing when exudate is within 1 cm of dressing edge.
- *Cavi care*®: conforming cavity dressing for deep, uninfected wounds.
- *Allevyn cavity wound dressing*®: foam chippings in a perforated film.

Hydrocolloids

- Made from cellulose, gelatin, and pectins to absorb water and form a gel, providing a moist environment
- Backing of vapour-permeable polyurethane film or foam
- Some are available as a paste
- Some have a wide adhesive border
- Suitable for granulating wounds with a low to moderate exudate, including surgical wounds, pressure sores, leg ulcers, and minor burns
- Promote rehydration and autolytic débridement of dry, sloughy, or necrotic wounds
- Manage blisters
- Impermeability to water allows bathing and showering with the dressing in place.
- Should be left in place for 4–5 days provided there is no infection.

Contraindications

- Infected wounds
- Patients with a hypersensitivity to hydrocolloid or its constituents

Problems

- Adhesion can be a problem, with the sides of the dressing rolling. To avoid:
  - allow a 2 cm overlap from the wound margin to the side of the dressing.
  - cover the dressing with an adhesive retention sheet if movement is likely to dislodge.
  - warm the dressing with the hands, preserving asepsis, prior to use.
  - ask the patient not to put weight on the area for 20 min, to allow the adhesion to be maximized.[1]

Hydrogels

- Made from co-polymer starch.
- Capable of significant fluid retention.
- Two types, amorphous and sheet:
  - *amorphous hydrogels* have no firm structure, their viscosity reduces as moisture is absorbed, e.g. Intrasite Gel®.
  - *sheet hydrogels*: structure is retained as fluid is absorbed, e.g. Geliperm®.
- Used for dry, sloughy, lightly exudating, granulating, or necrotic wounds.
- Can be used as a carrier for metronidazole for smelly fungating wounds.
- Apply a thick layer of gel followed by a secondary dressing when using an amorphous hydrogel.
- A secondary dressing is also required when using a sheet hydrogel.
- Secondary dressings: perforated plastic film, followed by an absorbent pad if heavy exudates; a vapour-permeable film dressing if little exudate.
- Dressings need to be changed every 3–4 days or daily when used with a dry wound.

1 Bux M (1996). Selection and use of wound dressings. *Wound Care for Pharmacists.* Summer issue 11–16

Contraindications
- Infected or heavily exudating wounds.
- Allergic reaction to some preparations.
- Not for wounds that are infected with *Pseudomonas*.

Vapour-permeable films and membranes
- Vapour-permeable polyurethane film coated with a synthetic adhesive.
- Use for postoperative dressings, decubitus ulcers, stoma care, and to prevent skin breakdown.
- Use as secondary dressings over alginates and foams.
- Sometimes used to protect vulnerable skin from damage.
- They allow the passage of water vapour and oxygen but not of water or micro-organisms.
- Provide a moist healing environment.

Contraindications
Not suitable for large wounds with heavy exudate, as exudates may cause the adhesive edges to wrinkle and allow risk of bacterial entry.

Table 12.22 Suitable dressings for different wound types[2]

Wound type	Dressing property	Dressing type
Dry, necrotic wound	Moisture retentive	Hydrocolloids
		Hydrogels
Slough-covered wound	Moisture retentive	Hydrocolloids
	Absorptive	Hydrogels
	Perhaps: absorbs odour, antimicrobial	
Clean, exudating wound	Absorptive	Hydrocolloids
	Perhaps: absorbs odour; antimicrobial	Foams
		Alginates
		If exudates high:
		• knitted varicose primary dressing
		• paraffin gauze
Dry	Moisture retentive	Absorbent perforated plastic film or vapour-permeable adhesive film
	Low adherence	
	Thermal insulation	

2 BNF (2003–2005). London British Medical Association and the Royal Pharmaceutical Society of Great Britain. London.

Types of preparations

Emollients

- Used to treat dry and scaling skin.
- Soothe and hydrate skin.
- Preparations with high water content produce the greater cooling effect on the skin (suitable for those suffering pruritis).
- A preparation with high oil content will help those with severely dry skin by sealing the skin and preventing further water loss.
- Should be applied in the direction of hair growth.

Creams

- Oil in water emulsions.
- Two actions:
  - first, water is lost from the cream by evaporation and absorption by the skin which it cools.
  - secondly, the water loss from the emulsion, added to the mechanical action of applying the mixture, releases the oils onto.
  - the surface of the skin, preventing further water loss.
- An example is aqueous cream a light emollient.

Ointments

- Greasy preparations commonly using a base of soft paraffin or a combination of soft, liquid, and hard paraffin.
- They do not normally contain water.
- More occlusive than creams.
- Effective for chronic dry lesions.
- An example is emulsifying ointment.

Contraindications

Sensitivity to hydrous wool fat (lanolin) should be suspected if a reaction occurs.

Both aqueous cream and emulsifying ointment can be used as a soap substitute.

Corticosteroids

- Hormones found in the cortex of the adrenal glands:
  - mineralocorticoids control the balance between water and mineral content of the body.
  - glucocorticoids help maintain the normal blood glucose, to assist the body in times of stress and injury.
- Large amounts of corticosteroids suppress the auto-immune system and this anti-inflammatory effect is the reason for their use.
- They act by inhibiting the enzymes that stimulate the formation of prostaglandin and leukotriene, to suppress the allergic/immune and inflammatory responses.

Adverse effects

- Mild and moderately potent topical corticosteroids are rarely associated with adverse effects.

- However, systemic absorption is increased if:
  - they are applied over a wide area
  - the skin is damaged
  - covered by an occlusive dressing.
- If the treatment is long term, systemic, and high dose, the following can occur:
  - hyperglycaemia
  - protein catabolism, leading to loss of bone mass, muscle atrophy, and thin skin
  - lipolysis, which can lead to Cushing's syndrome: 'moon face' or 'buffalo hump'
  - lessening of resistance to infection
  - poor wound healing
  - oedema
  - increased BP
  - sodium and water retention
  - hypokalemia
  - hirsutism
  - allergic reactions
  - increased gastric acidity.
- Always start on the least potent preparations and work up.

Table 12.23 Preparation potency of corticosteroids

Potency	Preparation
Mildly potent	Hydrocortisone
Moderately	Alclometasone
	Clobetasone
	Fluocinonide
	Fluocortolone
	Flurandrenolone
	Halcinonide
Potent	Beclomethasone
	Betamethasone
	Diflucortolone
	Desoxymethasone
	Flucinonide
	Fluticasone
	Mometasone
	Triamcinolone
Very potent	Halcinonide
	Clobetasol

Substance misuse and dependency

Background: controlled drugs

These are preparations that are subject to the Misuse of Drugs Regulations 2001 (see below) and are specified in schedules 2 and 3.

Principal legal requirements include a prescription which is:
- signed
- dated
- indelibly written and includes:
  - patient's name and address
  - the case, form, and strength of the preparation
  - total quantity of the preparation, or number of dose units in both words and figures
  - the dose
  - if issued by a dentist, the words 'for dental treatment only'.
- Prescribing and the law.

Drugs and substances of abuse and dependence

- Cocaine
- Diamorphine (heroin)
- Morphine
- Synthetic opioids
- Amphetamines
- Flunitrazepam
- Temazepam
- Barbiturates
- Cannabis
- Lysergide (LSD)
- 3,4-methylenedioxymetamphetamine (MDMA, ecstasy)
- Solvents and glue
- Petrol
- Antifreeze
- Alcohol
- Nicotine.

Misuse of drugs act 1971

This act prohibits the manufacture, supply, and possession of 'controlled drugs' except under due authority. Drugs are classified according to the degree of harm their misuse may cause.

Class A
- Alfentanil
- Cocaine
- Dextromoramide
- Diamorphine (heroin)
- Dipipanone
- Lysergide (LSD)
- Methadone
- MDMA
- Morphine
- Opium
- Pethidine
- Phencyclidine
- Remifentanil
- And all class B drugs prepared for injection.

Class B
- Oral amphetamines
- Barbiturates
- Cannabis
- Cannabis resin
- Codeine
- Ethylmorphine
- Glutethimide
- Pentazocine
- Phenmetrazine
- Pholcodine.

Class C
- Certain drugs related to amphetamines
- Buprenorphine
- Diethylpropion
- Mazindol
- Meprobamate
- Pemoline
- Pipradrol
- Most benzodiazepines
- Androgenic and anabolic steroids
- Clembutarol
- human Chorionic Gonadotrophin (hCG)
- Non-human chorionic gonadotrophin
- Somatrophin/somatropin
- Somatrem.

Misuse of Drugs Regulation 2001

Misuse of Drugs Regulations 2001

This defines the classes of person who are authorized to supply and possess controlled drugs while acting in their professional capacity. It also regulates the conditions under which these actions may be carried out.

Drugs are divided into five schedules specifying the import, export, production, supply, possession, prescribing, and record-keeping requirements. Examples of drugs under each schedule (see current BNF) are:

Schedule 1
- Cannabis.
- Lysergide.

These drugs may not be prescribed or possessed except in accordance with Home Office Authority.

Schedule 2
- Diamorphine (heroin)
- Morphine
- Remifentanil
- Pethidine
- Secobarbital
- Amphetamines
- Cocaine.

Schedule 3
- Barbiturates (except secobarbital, see schedule 2)
- Buprenorphine
- Diethylpropion
- Flunitrazepam
- Mazindol
- Meprobamate
- Pentazocine
- Phentermine
- Temazepam.

Schedule 4
- Some benzodiazepines
- Androgenic and anabolic steroids
- human Chorionic Gonadotrophin (hCG)
- Non-human chorionic gonadotrophin
- Somatrophin/somatropin
- Somatrem.

Schedule 5
Preparations of controlled drugs that are exempt from all controlled drug requirements, except the retention of invoices, for 2 years.

Background: statistics on drug misuse in young people aged under 25, in 1998

11–15-year-olds in England during the previous year
- 11% had used drugs in the previous year.
- Cannabis was the most commonly used illicit drug for this age group (10% of the sample).
- Amphetamines 2%.
- 2% poppers (amyl nitrate).
- 1% cocaine.
- <0.5% crack (a cocaine derivative) or heroin.

11–15-year-olds in England during the previous month
7% had used drugs.

16–24-year-olds
- 29% had used drugs—this level has been the same for 1994, 1996, and 1998.
- 27% had used cannabis in the preceding year.
- 10% amphetamines.
- 5% ecstasy.
- 5% poppers.
- 3% cocaine (use of this drug has increased from 1% in 1994).
- <0.5% crack or heroin.

The government's 10-year strategy for reducing drug misuse (*Tackling Drugs to Build a Better Britain*) seeks to move the emphasis from reactive rehabilitation to prevention. To help with this a drug prevention resource pack has been available since 2003

Further to this, in 2005 a briefing on nurse prescribing in substance misuse was published by the National Treatment Agency for Substance Misuse.

🖳 www.doh.uk.substance misuse.

Nicotine replacement therapy as an aid for smoking cessation

Tobacco smoke contains over 300 chemical compounds, including irritants such as tars, nicotine, and carbon monoxide, which are responsible for causing both short- and long-term effects.

Long-term effects
- coronary heart disease
- peripheral vascular disease (PVD)
- cerebrovascular disease
- lung cancer
- peptic ulceration
- chronic obstructive pulmonary disease (COPD)
- low birth weight at term for babies of mothers who smoked during their pregnancy.

Short-term effects
- emotional dependence on nicotine
- decreased removal of secretions from the lung as the cilia lining the bronchi are less active
- the oxygen-carrying capacity of the blood is reduced as there is an increase in carboxyhaemoglobin
- loss of appetite.

Nicotine
This agonist acts on receptors in the CNS to cause neuronal excitement, resulting in:
- tolerance
- physical dependence
- psychological dependence (cravings) and it is highly addictive.

Withdrawal symptoms include:
- the need to smoke tobacco
- depression
- irritability
- insomnia
- difficulty in concentration
- restlessness
- increased appetite, resulting in weight gain.

Smoking cessation interventions have proved to be a cost-effective way of preserving health and reducing ill-health caused by smoking tobacco.

Nicotine replacement therapy is useful to aid smoking cessation in those who smoke more than 10 cigarettes a day and its efficacy is enhanced if combined with behavioral support.

📖 Prescribing for public health.

Prescribing for the urinary system

Brief description of the urinary system

Structure of the urinary system comprises
- kidneys (usually two)
- paired ureters
- bladder
- urethra.

Urine drains from the kidneys at a rate of about 1 ml/min.

Kidneys
- Each kidney is the size of a fist and is supplied with blood via the renal arteries and veins.
- It can be considered as having three regions: the pelvis (transferring waste products from the medulla to the ureters), cortex (the outer covering), and medulla.
- There are about 225 km of fine blood vessels in each kidney. The filtration of blood to remove waste products takes place in glomeruli which contain Bowman's capsules and glomerular capillaries and are situated in the medulla region of the kidney.
- In addition to glomerular filtration to remove waste products, the kidneys also have a role in the control of blood pressure, maintenance of the acid–base balance of the blood, hormone production and synthesis of vitamin D.

Ureters
There are two ureters that carry urine from the pelvis of the kidneys to the bladder.

Bladder
- The bladder is a hollow, muscular organ with three orifices in its wall (openings to the two ureters and the urethra). It acts as a reservoir for urine, up to 600 ml between voidings, and expels urine at micturition.
- It is supported by the pelvic floor and two groups of muscles.
- The bladder wall comprises four layers:
  - the peritoneum, (covering the surface of the bladder)
  - the detrusor muscle.
  - the submucosa
  - the mucosa.

A child's bladder capacity can be calculated using:

Bladder capacity in ml = (age in years × 30) + 30

Urethra
- This forms a conduit to take urine from the bladder to the meatus.
In females it is about 4 cm long and has an external sphincter. In males it is about 20 cm long with both an external and internal sphincter.

📖 Prescribing for sexual health.

Function of the urinary system

- Excretion: removal of waste products from body fluids is one of the functions of the kidney.
- Elimination: removal to outside the body.

The vital functions of the urinary system are performed by the kidneys; however, problems with any of the conduction systems have an effect on renal function.

📖 Prescribing for renal disease.

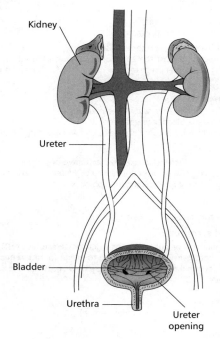

Fig. 12.7 Brief description of the urinary system. Reproduced from Glasper, EA, McEwing, G, Richardson, J. *Oxford Handbook of Children's and Young People's Nursing*, by kind permission of Oxford University Press.

Uncomplicated lower urinary tract infection (UTI) in women

Patient has an infection of their otherwise anatomically and physiologically normal urinary tract, with normal renal function and no associated illness to impair their defence mechanisms.

Risk factors

- Sexual intercourse
- Family history of UTI
- Use of a contraceptive diaphragm
- More common during pregnancy.

As women have a short urethra, close to both vagina and rectum, there is little protection against the entry of micro-organisms into the bladder. Normal changes during pregnancy predispose towards infection.

Prevention

- Adequate fluid intake
- Empty the bladder after sexual intercourse
- Don't allow the bladder to get overfull
- Ensure the bladder is completely emptied when passing urine.

Causes

- In 70% of cases *Escherichia coli* is the causative organism.
- The remaining 30% of cases are caused by *Proteus mirabilis*, *Klebsiella pneumonia*, and *Staphylococcus saprophyticus*.

Assessment

Patient's history and clinical signs.

Signs and symptoms

- Positive dipstick for pus in the urine (leucocyte esterase test) or for bacteria that alter nitrate in the urine to nitrite (nitrate reductase test)
- Lower abdominal discomfort; burning pain on passing urine
- Frequency
- Urgency
- Cloudy or foul-smelling urine
- Confusion (especially in the older person)
- Dysuria
- Haematuria.

Treatment

- Patients should drink 3 litres of fluid a day.
- Give sodium bicarbonate or potassium citrate to make the urine more alkaline and reduce the burning sensation on voiding.
- Cranberry products are recommended.[1,2]

1 Avorn J et al. (1994). Reduction of bacteriuria and pyuria after ingestion of cranberry juice. *JAMA*, **271**, 751–4.
2 Eichhorts AM et al. (1997). The therapeutic value of cranberries in treating and preventing urinary tract infections. *The Online Journal of Knowledge Synthesis in Nursing*, **4**, 2.

- Oral antibiotics may be prescribed (see current BNF for full list e.g. cefalexin or trimethoprim).
- Treat all UTIs during pregnancy and confirm cessation of the infection by urine sample culture.
- Mild analgesia or hot pads for localized pain relief.

Catheter patency problems

Patients with indwelling catheters are prone to patency problems such as blockage, catheter encrustation, inflammatory reactions, trauma, bladder infections, pain, and discomfort.
- 50% of patients have blockages secondary to encrustation.
- *Proteus, Klebsiella,* and *Pseudomonas* bacteria specifically facilitate the process of encrustation by providing urease enzymes that release ammonia and hydrogen ions from the urine, increasing its alkalinity.
- Micro-organisms also collect on the surface of the catheter, producing a biofilm that produces a glycocalyx (a thick coat of polysaccharides).

Risk factors
After 14 days, silicone-coated, Teflon®-coated and latex catheters are more likely to become encrusted than all-silicone catheters.[1]

Prevention
- Hydrogel-coated and all-silicone catheters appear to be resistant to encrustation for up to 18 weeks.
- Hydrogel-coated catheters are more resistant to biofilm than silicone-coated ones.
- It is possible to predict the length of time a catheter will last for individual patients by observing patterns of catheter life for each patient, thus preventing blockages by replacing catheters in time.
- Reducing urine alkalinity by consumption of cranberry juice may prolong catheter patency and prevent infection.
- Hydrogel-coated, all-silicone and silicone catheters require changing every 3 months to avoid blockage.
- Latex catheters require changing every 6 weeks.

Treatment
Blocked catheters require either changing (often painful for the patient) or washing out.
- Warm catheter patency solutions to body temperature.
- This is performed using aseptic technique.
- Encourage patients to maintain adequate fluid intake to keep urine dilute.
- Suggest that patients try cranberry products.

1 Winn, C. (1998). Complications with urinary catheters. *Professional Nurse*, **13**(5), S7–S10.

Urinary incontinence

An involuntary or inappropriate loss of urine which can be demonstrated objectively.[1] It may be classified into six categories, although they are not mutually exclusive:

Urge incontinence

This is caused by instability of the detrusor muscle, or hyperreflexia, which causes the bladder to contract at times other than intended urination. The bladder may not empty completely and a residual volume greater than 100 ml is common. The cause is unknown but it may be due to obstruction or neurological disease.

Overflow incontinence

The bladder overfills and urine leaks into the ureter. Symptoms include, voiding small amounts of urine, hesitancy, poor flow, or post-micturition dribble. This condition may follow hysterectomy or be caused by faecal impaction, unwanted effects of a drug regime, or prostatic hyperplasia.

Stress incontinence

An involuntary urine leak when abdominal pressure increases during physical activity, e.g. exercise or coughing. It is usually caused by muscular damage to the bladder outlet because of weakness of the pelvic floor musculature. Often precipitated by childbirth, post-menopausal oestrogen deficiency or as a complication following prostatic surgery.

Neuropathic bladder disorder

Caused by injury or disease of neuronal control which results in dysfunction of the lower urinary tract. Often associated with open or closed spina bifida, spinal chord tumour, trauma, and transverse myelitis.

Post-micturition dribble

Slight incontinence following micturition in males as the bulbo spongiosum muscle fails to evacuate the distal bulb of the urethra.

Functional incontinence

Despite a healthy and normal urinary tract, inappropriate voiding occurs due to environmental factors such as inaccessible toilets, impaired mobility.

Following assessment, which includes

- full symptom and medical history
- holistic needs assessment
- baseline assessment including mid-stream urine (MSU)
- discussion of patient's perception of the problem
- accurate diagnosis may be made and appropriate treatment decided, guided by local formularies and patient choice.

---

1 National Prescribing Center (1999). *Nurse prescribing resource pack—urinary incontinence*. NPC

Resources

The Continent Products Directory, Continence Foundation, 307 Hatton Square, 16 Baldwin Gardens, London EC 19 7RJ 🖳 www.vois.org.uk/cf

Local continence advisor phone number

PromoCon 2001 (Promoting continence through Product awareness), Disabled Living, Redbank House, 4 St Chad's Street, Cheetham, Manchester M8 8QA. ☎ Product helpline: 0161 834 2001

MDA: 🖳 www.medical-devices.gov.uk

Prescribing for sexual health

Brief overview of the female reproductive system

Structure and function

Ovaries (female gonads)

The ovaries are suspended, by the mesovarium, suspensory and ovarian ligaments, either side of the pelvis within the peritoneal cavity.

Ovaries produce oestrogen (Table 12.24), a hormone that stimulates the production and maturation of follicles which ripen to produce ova. This process is called oogenesis and occurs every 28 days between puberty and menopause.

Follicle stimulating hormone (FSH) and luteinizing hormone (LH), secreted by the hypothalamus, situated in the anterior lobe of the pituitary gland, control the menstrual cycle. This cycle facilitates the release of a mature ovum each month and prepares the lining of the uterus to receive and implant the fertilized ovum.

Fallopian or ovarian tubes

These muscular tubes, approximately 12 cm in length, are the conduit for the ripened ova between the ovary and uterus.

The widest part of the tube is proximate to the ovary and is called the infundibulum. This has a number of finger-like projections, called fimbriae, which waft fluid from the peritoneal cavity into the tube. The lining of the tube contains cilia, and the combination of strong muscular contractions and beating of the cilia enables the ova to be transported along the tube to the uterus.

The tube also provides an environment full of nutrients for both the sperm (spermatozoa) and fertilized egg.

Uterus

This hollow, pear-shaped organ is situated leaning forward within the pelvis behind the bladder. It consists of the body, or corpus, and the cervix. It is supported and stabilized by a broad ligament, other suspensory ligaments, skeletal muscles, and the fascia of the pelvic floor.

The body (corpus)

The fundus of the body is situated at its junction with the Fallopian tubes. This part is comprised of muscle and myometrium which is lined with endometrium (glandular tissue). Part of this endometrial tissue is shed during menstruation. During pregnancy the endometrium deals with the physiological needs of the developing fetus.

The cervix

At the lower end of the uterus, this structure, which points towards the spine, extends into the vagina and forms a curved surface enclosing a central opening called the cervical os. The cervix consists of mainly connective tissue with a little muscle. Cervical glands are situated within the epithelial lining of the cervix.

The vagina

Comprising bundles of smooth muscles, this tube passes through the pelvic floor and perineum. When pelvic and peritoneal muscles contract, a sphincter is formed around the opening to the vagina. Nutrients, for the flora of bacteria in the vagina, and lubricating secretions are provided by cervical glands. These maintain an acidic environment which can affect the motility of spermatozoa.

The external genitalia

Contained within the vulva, the labia minora and majora and the clitoris comprise the female external genitalia. Surrounding the vaginal opening is an area rich in sebaceous, sweat and mucus-secreting glands. Anterior to the vulva and the pubic symphysis is a bulging area of adipose deposit, the mons pubis.

📖 Prescribing for public health.

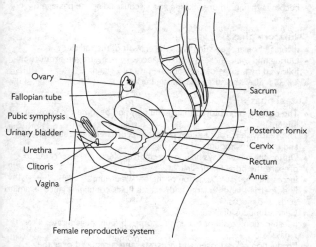

Ovary
Fallopian tube
Pubic symphysis
Urinary bladder
Urethra
Clitoris
Vagina

Sacrum
Uterus
Posterior fornix
Cervix
Rectum
Anus

Female reproductive system

Fig. 12.8 Brief overview of the female reproductive system. Reproduced from Glasper, EA, McEwing, G, Richardson, J. *Oxford Handbook of Children's and Young People's Nursing*, by kind permission of Oxford University Press.

The menstrual cycle

This can be divided into four phases:

Menstruaton

- Lasts for 4–6 days.
- Endometrium is shed and about 400 ml of blood is lost.
- Secretion of FSH and LH begin to increase, causing the maturation of several ovarian follicles.

Follicular phase

- On about day 6 of the cycle only one of the stimulated follicles continues to develop.
- Oestrogen production increases.
- Endometrium thickens.
- Cervical mucus throughout the vagina, uterus, and Fallopian tubes becomes thinner, more alkaline and viscous, aiding the passage of sperm.

Ovulatory phase

- Increased oestrogen stimulates the growth of the follicle.
- During mid cycle there is a further increase in oestrogen production followed by a surge of LH from the pituitary gland.
- 34–38 h after this surge the follicle bursts.

Luteal phase

- The cells of the ruptured follicle multiply and become the corpus luteum.
- The yellowish corpus luteum produces progesterone (Table 12.24) and moderate amounts of oestrogen.
- During the next 7 days high levels of progesterone are secreted to prepare the body for pregnancy.
- Increasing the vascularization of the endometrium.
- Endometrial glands enlarge and secrete fluids containing glucose, amino acids, and mucus.
- Cervical mucus thickens.
- If fertilization does not occur, the corpus luteum degenerates after 7 days.
- Production of oestrogen and progesterone is reduced over the 12 days following ovulation.
- Endometrial lining is shed.
- Oestrogen and progesterone are further reduced.
- FSH and LH begin a new cycle.

Fertilization

- Only one sperm normally fertilizes the ovum.
- The ovum travels to the uterus and implants in the endometrium.

Table 12.24 Main activities of oestrogen, progesterone, and progestogen

Hormone	Activity
Oestrogen	Development of sex hormone[LD1] in women
	Breast development
	Fat distribution
	Hair distribution
	During menstrual cycle[LD2]:
	Growth of endometrium
	Movement of fimbriae and contraction of uterine tube walls to enable passage of ovum
	Increase in sexual drive
	Thinning of cervical mucus
	Increased suppleness of vagina enabling it to expand during pregnancy, labour, and intercourse
	Water retention
	Stimulation of bone and muscle growth
	Stimulation of hepatic production of sex hormone binding globulin, HDLa and blood clotting factors
Progesterone	Continued preparation of the uterus for pregnancy
	In combination with prolactin, stimulates the breasts to produce milk
	Thickening of cervical mucus
Progestogen	Derived from testosterone; can stimulate excess hair growth and acne
	Increase in appetite and weight gain
	Reduction of sex drive
	Increased risk of CVD[LD3] by the reduction of HDL and an increase in LDL levels
	Reduction in sex hormone binding globulin
Sex hormone binding globulin	Reduces male characteristics
	Affects circulating testosterone and progestogens

a HDLs are complexes of lipid and protein which transport cholesterol away from peripheral tissue to the liver where they are stored or excreted in the bile.

Brief overview of the male reproductive system

Structure and function

The penis

When in flaccid state it is a soft cylinder of spongy tissue. Only ½ the length of the penis is visible outside the body.

The penis allows urine to be voided and the expulsion of spermatozoa during sexual intercourse or stimulation.

The penis has three main sections:

The root

This section attaches the penis to the underside of the pelvis.

The body

The tubular part of the penis, which comprises three cylindrical columns of erectile tissue, two corpora cavernosum and the corpus spongiosum.

The corpora cavernosa lie adjacent to each other and contain most of the erectile tissue of the penis. Within these structures are small spaces, the lacunar spaces, which are surrounded by smooth muscle. A tough fibrous coat, the tunica albicans, encases each of the corpora cavernoss.

The corpus spongiosum protects and surrounds the urethra on the underside of the penis. The tissue of the corpus spongiosum is erectile and the whole length expands during an erection. At the distal end the corpus spongiosum widens to form the glans or head of the penis.

The glans or head

This refers to the expanded distal end of the penis, which is surrounded by the prepuce or foreskin and contains the external urethral meatus.

The urethra

This has two functions, both to allow the voiding of urine from the bladder and to act as a channel for semen during ejaculation. A sphincter between the bladder and urethra contracts during ejaculation, preventing urine entering the urethra and sperm entering the bladder at this time.

The testicles (testes)

Two testicles are contained separately within the scrotum, a thin sack of skin and involuntary muscle, which hang on the outside of the body. This enables the testicles to be kept cool; in cold weather the involuntary muscle contracts and draws the scrotum nearer to the body to prevent overcooling. This muscular contraction also occurs in states of fear, anger, and sexual arousal.

The testicles produce and store spermatozoa and supply testosterone. This hormone is responsible for the production of male features such as facial hair, a deep voice, and the ability to have an erection.

The prostate

This is a walnut-sized gland which produces prostatic fluid a rich source of prostaglandin E, and accounts for 20% of semen volume.

📖 Prescribing for the endocrine system.

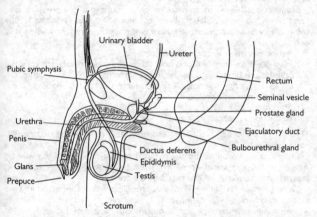

Fig. 12.9 Brief overview of the male reproductive system. Reproduced from Glasper, EA, McEwing, G, Richardson, J. *Oxford Handbook of Children's and Young People's Nursing*, by kind permission of Oxford University Press.

Erection emission and ejaculation

It is important to note that ejaculation and erection are two separate functions. A man can ejaculate from a flaccid penis and may have an erection without ejaculation

Erection is achieved by an increase of pressure in a low-pressure system. When the penis is flaccid it has less blood supplied (1/8th to 1/10th the erect penis volume), the pressure is therefore lower than when it is erect.

Erection has three important components:
(1) High-pressure arterial blood flow through the centre of each corpus cavernosum branching into the smaller arteries within the erectile tissue. These tiny arterioles leak blood into the lacunar spaces, causing the penis to expand.
(2) Smooth muscle relaxation,
(3) Reduction in venous drainage.

(1) and (2) are under autonomic and hormonal control; (3) occurs as a result of (1) and (2).

During sexual arousal the brain sends messages via parasympathetic nerves within the spinal cord, which cause smooth muscles to relax, arterial walls to dilate, and blood flow to increase.

During sexual activity sperm are propelled from the penis in two stages, emission and ejaculation:
• emission involves contraction of the smooth muscle of the vas deferens, seminal vesicles, and prostate gland, expelling semen into the urethra
• ejaculation is achieved by contraction of the striated muscle at the base of the penis which enables semen to be expelled from the penis.

During heterosexual intercourse, sperm reach the uterine tubes within hours of intercourse and ejaculation, although they are viable for up to 7 days. During this period they become more able to adhere to the ovum, which improves the facilitation of fertilization.

Contraception

For complete lists of generic named examples, interactions, contra-indications and side-effects please see the section on contraceptives in the BNF.

Emergency contraception

This can be either one of two oral hormonal preparations containing levonorgestrel or a copper-containing IUD.

Hormonal preparations
- Less effective than an IUD
- Efficacy deteriorates with time
- Effective if the dose is taken within 72 h (3 days) of unprotected intercourse.

IUD
- A copper IUD can be inserted up to 120 h (5 days) after unprotected sex.
- If more than 5 days since unprotected intercourse, the device will still be effective if inserted up to 5 days after the earliest calculated day when ovulation took place (that is before implantation).

WHO (1998)[1] considers established pregnancy as the only contraindication for any of these preparations.

Injected progestogens

These contain a higher dose than oral pills and have a similar effect. Almost 100% effective and given IM, protection lasts for 8 weeks; however, there may be a delayed return to fertility.

Implanted progestogens (Implanon®)

This single flexible rod may be inserted subdermally into the lower surface of the upper arm. Protection lasts for up to 3 years. Women with a body mass < 35 kg/m² may not be protected during the third year.

Intra-uterine devices (IUDs)

These devices are fitted into the uterus and consist of a plastic carrier with copper wire or copper bands. They are suitable for older women, and if fitted over the age of 40 may remain in place until after the menopause. Effectiveness ranges from 98 to almost 100%.

Mode of action
- IUDs produce an inflammatory reaction in the uterus.
- Leucocytes respond to this inflammatory condition and also destroy sperm and possibly the ova, also disrupting the endometrium and preventing implantation.
- Prostaglandins are stimulated by the presence of the IUD and these produce uterine contractions.
- Some IUDs, for example Mirena® release a low dose of progestogen, adding a similar effect to that of a POP.

1 WHO (1998). *Emergency contraceptions: A guide to service delivery.* WHO, Geneva.

Spermicides

- These need to be used in conjunction with barrier methods as their failure rate is high if used alone.
- They contain an active ingredient which destroys the sperm membrane and alters the pH of the vaginal environment, and need to be introduced into the vagina before intercourse.
- They are made in a variety of forms:
  - creams
  - foams
  - pessaries.

Combined oral hormonal contraception (COC)

This method of contraception is second only to sterilization: effectiveness ranging from 99.03% to 99.90%. Despite improvements over the 40 years since it was first used, it does have many unwanted side-effects, both minor and major.

Action of COCs
- COCs inhibit the action of FSH, suppressing follicular growth and the increase in levels of oestrogen.
- The surge in LH is not produced.
- Cervical mucus remains viscous and is no longer stretchy, impairing the transport and penetration of sperm.
- Sperm migration is further thwarted as the changes to motility and secretions within the uterine tubes do not take place.
- Implantation is prevented.

There are several different types of COC:
- *monophasic:* each tablet contains a fixed amount of oestrogen and progestogen. Tablets are taken orally for 21 consecutive days out of each 28-day cycle and withdrawal bleeding occurs during the 7 days they are not taken.
- *biphasic and triphasic:* these contain varying amounts of hormones depending on the stage of the cycle. They are taken for 21 of 28 days with a 7-day break.
- *everyday pill:* these may be monophasic, biphasic or triphasic and are taken for each of the 28 days. As some of the pills are inactive, it is essential to take them in the correct order.

Advantages of COCs
Include:
- reliable and reversible
- convenient
- menstruation predictable and regular
- reduces PMT
- lessens menorrhagia
- reduces dysmenorrhoea
- reduces the risk of benign breast disease, endometriosis, ectopic pregnancy, ovarian cysts, and endometrial and ovarian cancer
- less risk of PID than with intrauterine devices.

Disadvantages of COCs
Those with diabetes mellitus, family history of MI or CVA or are older, obese, or who smoke are at greater risk of the adverse effects of COCs. Disadvantages include:
- need to have a concordant agreement with the user
- risk of thromboembolism, heart disease, increase in BP, jaundice, gallstones, liver cancer
- risk of COC failing if taking broad-spectrum antibiotics so extra precautions are recomended.

Progesterone-only pill (POP)

POPs may be used if COCs are contraindicated as they contain the progestogens, norethisterone, etynodiol diacetate, or levonorgestrel. Although they have a higher failure rate, effectiveness ranges from 90 to 99%, they are suitable for older women, smokers, those with hypertension, heart valve disease, diabetes mellitus and migraine.

Action of POPs
- Possible prevention of ovulation.
- Thickening of cervical mucus, thereby impeding the transit of sperm.
- Thickening of endometrial lining of the uterus, which prevents implantation.

Advantages of POPs
Include:
- no increased risk of CVD, venous thrombolism, or hypertension
- can be continued prior to surgery
- are suitable for women who are breast feeding
- may reduce dysmenorrhoea and PMT.

Disadvantages of POPs
Include:
- each pill needs to be taken within 3 hours of the time of day that the previous day's pill was taken
- periods may no longer be regular
- can cause development of functional ovarian cysts
- slight risk of ectopic pregnancy
- same risk of breast cancer as COC.

Advice from the family planning organization regarding missed pills
'If your pill was more than three hours overdue you are not protected. Continue normal pill taking but use another form of contraceptive for the next 7 days.'

Barrier methods

Female barrier methods of contraception

These provide a barrier between the egg and sperm, thus preventing fertilization.

Diaphragm

- This is a dome-shaped cap made of latex rubber which is positioned in the vagina to cover the cervix.
- If used correctly with a spermicidal preparation, it is between 92% and 96% effective.
- There are three types of diaphragm:
  - **flat spring diaphragm:** this is used for women whose cervix is in the anterior or midplane position. It is between 55–95 mm in size and has a flat spring in the rim.
  - **coil spring diaphragm:** the spring in the rim of this device is coiled and women with a shallow symphysis pubis find this device more comfortable. It is between 55–100 mm in size.
  - **arching spring diaphragm:** women who have a cervix in the posterior position, or find it difficult to insert either of the other types, find this a useful alternative. It is between 65–95 mm in size.

Cap

The cap is smaller than the diaphragm and is made of rubber. It covers the cervix and is held in place by suction to the vaginal or cervical wall and is between 92–96% effective if used correctly with a spermicide. There are three types of cap:

- *vault cap:* semicircular, dome shaped and shallow; 55–75 mm in size.
- *cervical cap:* thimble-shaped with a firm rim; sizes range from 22 to 31 mm. Useful for women with a symmetrical cervix.
- *vimule cap:* a combination of the vault and cervical, it can be used by women with an irregularly shaped cervix. Sizes range between 42, 48, and 55 mm.

Male barrier methods of contraception

The condom or sheath

These latex coverings for the erect penis retain the sperm at ejaculation and prevent its entering the vagina. They should be used with a spermicide and are available in a number of styles, sizes, and finishes.

📖 Prescribing for public health.

---

1 WHO (1998). Emergency contraception: A guide to service delivery. WHO, Geneva.

Common conditions

Bacterial vaginosis

Bacterial infection of the vagina; only 50% of women with this infection report symptoms.

Cause

- The most common cause is an alteration in the normal flora of the vagina, from a predominance of *Lactobacillus* to a high concentration of anaerobic bacteria.
- It has been identified that the incidence of bacterial vaginosis is increased in women using IUDs and those taking oral contraceptives.
- Other risk factors include new or multiple sexual partners, sexual debut at a young age, and douching.[1]

Treatment

- Clindamycin cream 2% (Dalacin® cream)
- Metronidazole vaginal gel 0.75% (Zidival® vaginal gel)
- Metronidazole PO

Vulvovaginal candidiasis (thrush)

Cause

This inflammation is usually caused by a yeast, *Candida albicans*.

Signs and symptoms

Vulval itching and soreness; vaginal discharge; pain during intercourse.

Treatment: all partners

GI in BNF for imidazole preparations, which are formulated as pessaries, capsules, or intravaginal creams.

📖 Prescribing for infections

Dysmenorrhoea

Lower abdominal or pelvic pain experienced during menstruation.

Treatment

To control the pain with minimal side effects (📖 Prescribing for pain).
- NSAIDs have been used beneficially (e.g. mefenamic acid).

Balanitis

An inflammation of the glans penis.

Cause

Usually caused by bacterial or fungal infections and often associated with phimosis, an inability to retract the foreskin.

Signs and symptoms

Redness, itch, discharge

Treatment

As vulvovaginal candidiasis, with imidazoles or antifungals such as nystatin.

1 CEG (1999). *National Guidelines on the management of bacterial vaginosis*. Clinical Effectiveness group of the Association for Genitourinary Medicine and the Medical society for the study of Venereal disease. 🖳 www.agum.org.uk/CEG/S16

Prescribing for palliative care

Prescribing for palliative care

Definition

Prescribing for people who require palliative care involves the active total care and suppression of symptoms for those whose disease is not responsive to curative treatments. In addition to control of pain and other symptoms, it involves an holistic approach, embracing social, psychological, and spiritual dimensions.

Support is required for both the patient and the family and/or carers if quality of life is to be optimized for the patient.

Care is provided by a multidisciplinary team and may be delivered in the patient's home, at a day hospice, or an in-patient hospice.

Palliative care may be required by patients:
- who have cancer
- with debilitating progressive illness, such as heart failure
- with multiple sclerosis, motor neuron disease, or HIV/AIDS.

Treatment

The number of drugs should be limited to as few as possible, as taking oral medication can be an effort.

The approach required for prescribing by members of a multidisciplinary team requires liaison between the professionals involved. Communication and record keeping are key to ensure all medications prescribed are compatible with each other and the possible multipathology of the patient.

📖 7 principles of safe prescribing.

Provided the patient is not suffering from nausea, dysphagia, vomiting, or coma, oral medications are usually satisfactory.

Negotiating a contract

As with all prescribing, it is important to reach a concordant agreement with your patient (📖 Concordance; 📖 Prescribing pyramid). However, in addition to the recognition and treatment of symptoms identified through assessment and examination, it is important to consider:
- patient preference and concordance
- patient perception of severity of symptoms
- quality of life issues
- value for money considerations
- the roles of other members of the multidisciplinary team.

📖 Concordance.
📖 To ensure an effective consultation.

Management of anxiety

Definition
A universally unpleasant emotion than can be acute/transient or chronic/persistent.[1]

Possible causes for people requiring management of anxiety
- Situational
- Organic
- Psychiatric
- Drug induced
- Spiritual.

Symptoms and signs
- Poor concentration
- Indecisiveness
- Insomnia
- Irritability
- Sweating
- Tremor
- Panic attacks.

Treatment
Benzodiazepines.

1 Twycross, R. (1997). *Symptom management in advanced cancer*, (2nd edn). Radcliffe Medical Press, Abingdon.

Table 12.25 Drugs that may affect renal and hepatic function (adapted from the Joint Formulary Committee 2002)[2]

Area	Drug name	Symptom control
Renal	Aspirin	Pain
	Baclofen	Muscle spasm
	Cimetidine	Gastric hyperacidity
	Domperidone	Nausea and vomiting
	Famotidine	Gastric hyperacidity
	Ibuprofen	Mild to moderate pain
	Metoclopramide	Nausea and vomiting
	Ranitidine	Gastric hyperacidity
Hepatic	Aspirin	Mild to moderate pain
	Cimetidine	Gastric hyperacidity
	Cyclizine	Nausea and vomiting
	Dantrolene	Muscle spasm
	Diclofenac	Pain (NSAID external use)
	Ibuprofen	Pain (NSAID)
	Ketoprofen	Pain (NSAID external use)
	Metoclopramide	Nausea and vomiting
	Metronidazole	Fungating wounds
	Miconazole	Oral candidiasis (local)
	Paracetamol	Pain
	Ranitidine	Gastric hyperacidity

2 Joint Formulary Committee (2002). *British National Formulary* 44. British Medical Association and Royal Pharmaceutical Association of Great Britain, London.

Management of pain

See also Table 12.25 in 📖 Management of anxiety.
📖 Prescribing for pain.
📖 Prescribing for people with renal disease.

Opioids

- If non-opioids prove insufficient for mild to moderate pain control, opioids such as codeine and dextropropoxyphene may be given alone or in combination with non-opioids.
- Tramadol may be useful for moderate pain.
- Morphine is the most useful opiate if the above are failing to control pain (Fig. 12.10).
- Morphine often causes nausea and vomiting in adults and may need to be given with an anti-emetic.
- Other unwanted effects of morphine use include drowsiness and constipation.
- Larger doses may cause respiratory depression and hypotension.
- Consideration of possible dependence is not a deterrent for use of morphine in terminal illness.
- Patients are often prescribed morphine tablets in slow-release formulation as a form of pain control in palliative care.
- Alongside of this they may be presciced non-slow-release morphine to take when their pain is not controlled by the slow-release formulation, sometimes called a 'rescue dose'.
- The active life of non-slow-release morphine is around 4 h and it can be administered up to six times daily.
- A rescue dose may be needed 30 min or so before activity which causes pain, for example a wound redressing.

Breakthrough pain

Formula for calculating morphine dose for breakthrough pain*:

Breakthrough dose = (total daily dose of slow-release morphine)/6

e.g. 120 mg (slow-release morphine) × 2/6 = 40 mg

*Changing patients from oral morphine to diamorphine via a syringe driver (see table in BNF 'Prescribing in Palliative Care').

*Changing from oral morphine to fentanyl patch (slow-release dose over 3 days) (see BNF 7.2 and 'Prescribing in Palliative Care').

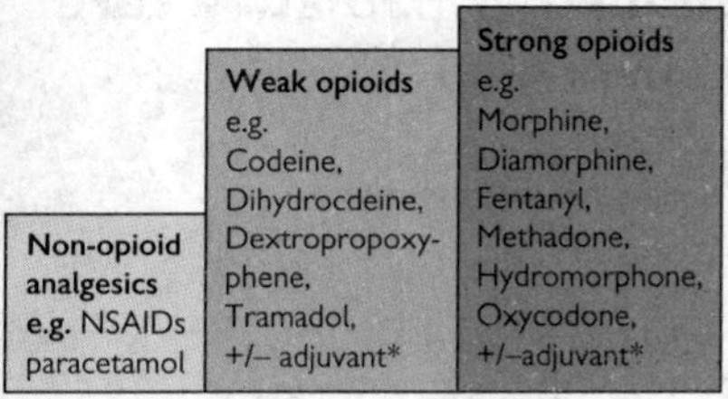

Fig. 12.10 WHO analgesic ladder.[1] *Adjuvant analgesics are drugs that have a primary indication which is not pain but can potentiate or enhance the effect of opioids, can treat the symptoms of the pain, or can help balance the doses to minimize the dose-related unwanted effects of opioids.

1 World Health Organization (1986). *Cancer pain relief*. WHO, Geneva.

Management of further palliative care related conditions (A–Z)

Constipation

Possible causes for people requiring palliative care

- Stress
- Diet or lack of
- Lack of exercise
- Reduced fluid intake
- Medication
- Underlying disease process.

For treatment, see 📖 Constipation.

Cough

This may be a symptom of an underlying pathology, asthma or post nasal drip, for example, and prescribing must follow assessment of the causes.

Morphine is the drug of choice for cough,[1] although the unwanted effects of sputum retention and ventilatory failure may contraindicate its use.

Diarrhoea

Possible causes for people requiring palliative care

- Excessive use of laxatives, antibiotics, antacids
- Infection
- Fistula
- Anxiety
- Irritable bowel
- Neurological dysfunction
- Autonomic insufficiency.

Dry mouth

Establish the cause, which could be dehydration, infection, anxiety or an unwanted effect of a medication, and resolve if possible.

Excessive respiratory secretions

The Joint Formulary Committee (2002)[1] has recommended the use of hyocine hydrobromide although it can cause agitation. It notes that hyocine butylbromide has fewer unwanted side effects but it is less effective in controlling these secretions.

Fungating wounds

Wound care products that contain charcoal may be useful when dressing these often malodorous wounds. See Table 12.22 📖 Types of dressing.

Gastric hyperactivity

(See Table 12.25 📖 Management of anxiety.)

It should be noted that H_2-receptor antagonists, which are useful for this symptom, do not protect against ulceration caused by NSAIDs which are commonly prescribed for pain relief in patients requiring palliative care.

Muscle spasm

(see Table 12.25 📖 Management of anxiety.)

Possible causes for people requiring palliative care

- Drug induced
- Meningeal metaseses
- Bone metastases
- Nerve compression
- Peripheral neuropathy
- Polymyostis
- Spinal degeneration.

Treatment

- Relaxation and massage techniques.
- Muscle relaxants such as diazepam or baclofen which inhibit nerve transmission through the spinal column and depress the CNS response.

Nausea and vomiting

Care consists of the management of symptoms. It is important to remember that oral anti-emetics will not be absorbed if there is gastric stasis.

Oral candidiasis

60% of patients with cancer have oral problems: either dry mouth or candida.

📖 Prescribing for gastrointestinal problems.

Restlessness, agitation, and confusion

Possible causes for people requiring palliative care

- Cognitive impairment
- Drug reaction.

Treatment

Phenothiazines such as levomepromazine and antipsychotic (neuroleptic) preparations.

Further information

For further information beyond the scope of this handbook.
🖳 www.macmillan.org.uk
🖳 www.cancerresearchuk.org/aboutcancer.
National Cancer Institute: 🖳 www.cancer.gov/cancerinfo/pdq/supportivecare
National Council for Hospice and Specialist Palliative Care Services (NCHSPCS): 🖳 www.hospice-spec-council.org.uk/

Cancer helplines

Cancer BACUP ☎ 0808001234
CancerHelp UK 🖳 www.cancerhelp.org.uk
Everyman Campaign 🖳 www.icr.ac.uk/everyman

Complementary and alternative medicines and over the counter drugs

Complementary and alternative medicines (CAMs)

What are CAMs?

- Complementary and alternative medicines. The treatment of disease using methods other than recognized/conventional medicine.
- Use of homeopathic, herbal, aromatherapy, and over the counter (OTC) vitamin supplements to treat conditions.

Problems

- Often not adequately clinically trialled.
- Might not have a product licence.
- Poor manufacturing process.
- Adulteration to include toxic substances and conventional drugs.
- Misidentification of herbs.
- Substitution of herbs.
- Varying strengths of preparations.
- Incomplete labelling.
- Incorrect dosage and instructions.
- Patients may see treatments/medications as 'natural' and not inform their health professional that they are taking them.
- Information not readily available in 'conventional' textbooks.

When prescribing

- Always ask the patient what else they are taking including OTC medication and herbal medicines.
- Consider potential drug interactions[1,2].

History

- At least 5,000 years old.
- Interest in CAMs has grown over past two decades.
- Over 31 million visits to CAM practitioners in 1998[3].
- One in five Britons seeks complementary or alternative therapy.
- Perceived to be 'safe'.
- Research lagging behind.
- Health care professionals are thought to know about it.

House of Lords Select Committee 2000 (recommendations)

- Tougher regulation.
- More rigorous testing.
- Greater supervision of practice.
- Only those with a statutory regulation or powerful self-regulation should be available on NHS.
- Only by referral from GP.

1 British Medical Association and Royal Pharmaceutical Society of Great Britain. *British National Formulary* (current edition). London.

2 Stockley, I. H. (2002). *Drug interactions* (6th edn). Pharmaceutical Press. London.

3 Thomas, K, Nicholl J.P., and Coleman, P. (2001). Use and expenditure on complementary therapies in England: a population based survey. *Complementary Therapies in Medicine*, **9**(1), 2–11.

Homeopathic and herbal medicines

Homeopathic

- Homeopathy: homeos (similar) pathos (disease).
- Like cures like—the mild effects of the remedy mimics the symptom of the disease.
- The greater the dilution, the greater the therapeutic effect (serial dilution)—hardly any or no trace of active ingredient.
- Manufacture controlled by Medicines Act 1968.
- Medical claims cannot be made for remedies, however, leaflets can be displayed near to product.
- Medical homeopaths are medically qualified and regulated by General medical Council (GMC).
- Non medical homeopaths (regulated by different bodies/Fellowship of homeopaths etc.).

Effects on patients

- Limited evidence with regard to ADRs.
- Little evidence with regards to drug interactions.

Herbalism

Regulated by:

- National Institute of Medical Herbalists 1864 (professional body).
- phytotherapy—the science of herbalism.

Herbal medicines

- Plant derived medicines at pharmacological doses where effects can be measured.
- Symptom based approach to diagnosis.

Regulation of herbal medicines

- Licensed: marketing authorization (product licence) issued by Medicines and Health Care Products Regulatory Agency (MHRA).
- Have to meet safety, quality and efficacy standards similar to conventional drugs.
- Unlicensed: exempt from licensing requirements (Section 12 of Medicines Act 1968).

Section 12 Medicines Act 1968

- Section 12 (1): a person can make, sell, and supply herbal remedies as part of business provided remedy is manufactured on the premises and supplied as the consequence of a consultation between patient and herbalist
- 12(2): allows manufacture and supply where:
  - Process of manufacture consists of drying, crushing or comminuting.
  - Remedy sold without any written recommendation as to its use.
  - Remedy sold under a designation which only specifies the plant and the process and does not apply any other name to the remedy.
- 📖 Legal differences between prescribing.

Table 13.1 Commonly used herbal medicines

Name of drug	Indications	Side effects	Drug interactions	Cautions/contraindications
Gluco-samine	For relief of joint pain	Mild GI symptoms, rash, drowsiness, headache, insomnia		Diabetes may alter glucose sensitivity. Caution in breast feeding. Contra-indicated if allergic to shellfish
Saw palmetto	Urogenital conditions —benign prostatic hyperplasis	Dizziness and GI disturbance. Rare side effects are: mild puritus, headache and hypertension. erectile dysfunction (similar to placebo effect in studies)	Hormonal therapies (contraception and hormonal replacement therapy)	Cautions: pregnancy and breast feeding. hormone dependent cancers
Valerian	Insomnia	Headache, drowsiness (sedation) GI symptoms Rarely: nervous excitability, cardiac disturbances on sudden withdrawal (not confirmed in trials) Can cause dependency		Pregnancy and breastfeeding, before driving or operating heavy machinery Not to be taken if known hyper-sensitivity
St John's Wort	Mild depression		Liver enzyme inducer for anti-epileptics, theophylline, the combined contraception pill, SSRIs, warfarin	Avoid during pregnancy, breast feeding. Avoid when taking anti epileptics, theophyline, the combined contraceptive pill and when taking SSRIs or warfarin
Echinacea	Prevention of upper respiratory tract infections	Nausea, dizziness, shortness of breath, burning and numbing sensation of tongue, dermatitis, hepatitis, puritus, hepatotoxicity	Other hepato-toxic drugs, e.g. anabolic steroids, amiodarone, ketoconazole, and meth-otrexate also might decrease the effect of immuno suppressants	Cautions: asthma, atopy, allergy or hypersensitivity to sunflowers, liver dysfunction, TB, diabetes, HIV, Systemic Lupus, and other auto-immune diseases

Safety of homeopathic and herbal medicines

Safety should be considered due to:
- a lack of data
- 'natural' does not always mean safe e.g. digitalis
- remember herbal remedies are medicines
- report adverse reactions to doctor or pharmacist
- may interact with other medicines.

Alert
- Patients taking drugs with a narrow therapeutic index (e.g. warfarin) or a drug therapy which is considered critical (e.g. insulin) should avoid using complementary medicines.
- Women who are pregnant or breastfeeding should avoid complementary medicines.
- Kava-Kava now withdrawn from the market due to yellow card reporting of severe hepatotoxicity.
- Some Chinese medicines contain harmful excipients.
  📖 Basic priniciples of pharmacology.

Reporting
- To the Medicines and Healthcare Products Regulatory Agency (MHRA) using yellow card reporting.
- Important for all drugs especially those less well known.
  📖 Drug effects.

Further reading
Zollman, C., Vickers, A. (1999). ABC of complementary medicine: what is complementary medicine? *BMJ* **319**, 693–6.
📖http://www.mcs.gov.uk/ourwork/licensingmeds/herbalsafety
UKMI Complementary Medicines Summaries December 2002. 📖www.ukmi.nhs.uk

Other complementary therapies

Chiropractic
A form of health care which focuses on correcting spinal problems and the function of the nervous system without the use of drugs or surgery.

Professional or representative association:
British Chiropractic Association
 Contact e-mail: enquiries@chiropractic-uk.co.uk

Osteopathy
A system of health care which focuses on balancing the musculoskeletal system to prevent and treat disease
Professional or representative association: British Osteopathic Association.
 Website: www.osteopathy.org

Acupuncture
Originally based on the ancient Chinese technique of inserting thin needles at specific points in the body. Used to control pain and other symptoms.
Professional or representative association: British Acupuncture Council
 Website: www.acupuncture.org.uk

Reflexology
Based on the ancient Chinese technique to restore energy flow throughout the body by the application of pressure point massage (mainly the feet, but can be the hands and ears).
Professional or representative association: British Reflexology Association
 Website: www.britreflex.co.uk

Aromatherapy
Uses essential oils (either extracts or essences often in conjunction with massage) to prevent or to treat disease
Professional or representative association: British Council of practising aromatherapists
 Email: info@bcapa.org
Professional or representative association: Aromatherapy Organisations Council
 Website: www.aromatherapy-uk.org

Healing

Can be defined as natural or spiritual. The use of either hands on or no touch technique to restore the energy flow through the body to support the body's own healing mechanisms.

Professional or representative association: National Federation of Spiritual Healers

Website: www.nfsh.org.uk

Naturopathy

The use of natural agents to support the internal balance of the body, promoting health and well being

Professional or representative association: The British Naturopathic Association

Website: www.naturopaths.org.uk

Over the counter drugs (OTCs)

Background

The NHS Plan[1] places emphasis on encouraging a growth in self care by extending the range of medicines available over the counter. To facilitate this, many items which were formerly prescription only medicines (POMs) have been classified as pharmacy (P) or general sales list (GSL). It is acknowledged that this increase in the number of medications available OTC will not necessarily reduce the prescribing burden of either doctors or NPs. It is unlikely that patients with enduring conditions who do not currently pay for their prescriptions will elect to purchase them OTC.[2]

It is important to note that OTC licences may not mirror POM licences. E.g. hydrocortisone 1% cream sold OTC may not be used on the face. Before advising OTC purchases always be sure the licence permits the use required.

Responsibilities

- Prescribers are equally accountable whether they recommend an OTC drug or prescribe a product and it is important to bear in mind the Nursing and Midwifery Council (NMC) guidelines on prescribing.
- NPs need to be vigilant when taking a medication history to ensure patients tell them of all products they are taking, including OTCs and homely remedies.
- It may be helpful to set up local guidelines to ensure good communication between community pharmacists, GPs and non-medical prescribers to ensure the best use of OTC products for the benefit of patients.

📖 Nursing and Midwifery Council (NMC) Code of Professional Conduct

Possible problems

There are several problems engendered by the move to an extended availability of OTC products.

- Many patients may take OTC products and fail to inform their GP, giving rise to potential drug interactions.
- Direct advertising to the general public, which is permitted for an OTC product, may increase demand for the product as a prescribed item.
- Direct advertising may also lead to products being taken which are not required, or which are contraindicated by other medication being taken, either prescribed or OTC.
- Ethical issues of equity and fairness arise if a decision is made to recommend a product as an OTC to one patient whilst deciding to prescribe for another, even if the decision to prescribe is based on evidence that the patient would choose not to purchase the item even if essential.

---

1 Department of Health (2000). *The NHS Plan: A plan for investment. A plan for reform.* The Stationary Office, London.
2 Bellingham, C. (2002). To switch or not? Pharmacists' opinions. *Pharmaceutical Journal.* **268**,

Increasing the prescribing rights of nurse independent prescribers may increase the numbers of problems outlined above.

📖 Prescribing for GI.
📖 Ethical issues.
📖 Cost effective prescribing.

Section 4

Accountability

Parameters of nurse prescribing

Legal parameters of nurse prescribing

Nurse independent prescribers are able to prescribe (from Spring/ Summer 2006) drugs from anywhere within the BNF (with the inclusion of some controlled drugs) providing that they are prescribing within their field of competence and that the drugs carry a product licence. Supplementary prescribers can prescribe unlicensed drugs and drugs outside of their product licence and controlled drugs as part of an agreed clinical management plan.

Legal categories of drugs

Drugs and medicinal products are classified into three different categories
- Prescription only medicines (POMs) can only be prescribed by a qualified prescriber as a result of a written prescription.
- Pharmacy only medicines (P) medicines are sold over the counter to the patient on request by a registered pharmacist who works in a registered pharmacy.
- General sales list medicines (GSL) medicines can be sold to patients in shops such as supermarkets, corner shops, petrol stations, etc.

Testing new drugs

Once it has been developed in the laboratory, a new drug is tested in three phases.
- Phase one: testing on healthy human volunteers to assess pharmaco-kinetics and dynamics and immediate general safety e.g. toxicity.
- Phase two: tested on patients in small scale clinical trials. Used to assess efficacy of dose and dose range etc.
- Phase three: tested in large randomized and usually double blind clinical trials to assess comparative efficacy against other drugs and or against placebo.

Drug licensing

- The results of the clinical trial(s) in terms of safety and efficacy are presented to the Medicines and Health Care Regulatory Agency (MHRA) in the United Kingdom (UK) or to the European Medicines Evaluation Agency (EMEA) (All European States including the UK). The above bodies will consider the results and issue the product with a licence for:
  - specific clinical indications
  - routes of administration
  - dose ranges.

Unlicensed medication

This term refers to:
• medicinal products for which no product licence has been issued.

Drugs outside of product license

• medicinal products for which are being used for clinical indications, routes of administration and dose range which are outside of their product licence.

Licensing and special groups

Medicinal products are often not awarded a licence for special groups such as older people, children, and pregnant and breastfeeding, women. This is because of the ethical difficulties and safety issues which may arise when manufacturers apply to conduct clinical trials.
• When a new product is launched the licence is usually limited to specific indications, dose ranges, and routes of administration at the time of product launch.
• As evidence of safety and efficacy becomes apparent as a result of post marketing surveillance the indications, dose range, and routes of administration may be added to.
• Generic drugs are normally awarded the existing licence indications of the patented brand.

Prescribing unlicensed medication

• Only prescribe as a supplementary prescriber in agreement with the independent prescriber and with the knowledge and the informed consent of the patient.
• Be aware of research if any.
• Balance benefits against risks.

Working with the pharmaceutical industry

What is the pharmaceutical industry?

The pharmaceutical industry consists of independent profit making pharmaceutical companies who work in competition to invent, manufacture and provide existing tried and tested drugs for the treatment of medical conditions and to research and develop new drugs in order to advance the treatment of new conditions.

Employees of the pharmaceutical industry have their own code of conduct provided by the Association of British Pharmaceutical Industries (ABPI) which can be accessed by linking to the following web site. ▣ www.abpi.org.uk Not all pharmaceutical companies are members of the ABPI and some companies observe the code although they are not members. There is national guidance on 'Commercial Sponsorship: Ethical Standards for the NHS' at:

▣ http://www.dh.gov.uk/assetRoot/04/07/60/78/04076078.pdf

This guidance can be used to underpin local policies.

Support for prescribing

The pharmaceutical industry provides a positive contribution towards:
- the advancement of medical care
- government revenue
- educational development
- support for specialist nurses in care delivery.

When working with drug representatives/the drug industry

- Identify local policy and protocol with regard to conduct and adhere to these.
- View literature and evidence as provided by the industry with a critical analytical and comparative eye.
- Consider accessing a range of information sources to support decision-making.
- Challenge practice and be aware of the ABPI if code of conduct[1].
- Be aware of pressure to prescribe.
- Be aware of subliminal and overt advertising e.g. mugs and pens, advertisements in journals, stands at events, direct mailing, etc.
- Look for more information than is given in an advertisement.
- Ask for copies of published references on efficacy and safety and check their quality.
- Suggested good practice is to accept offers of visits from reps by appointment only.
- Take control of the discussion.
- Make sure you get all the information you need about the product, including the cost.
- Ask for a copy of the summary of product characteristics (SPC) which can also be obtained on 🖳 www.medicines.org.
- Consider references from credible peer-reviewed journals first.
- Check what specialists in the field know about the product.

Questions to ask pharmaceutical reps

- What is this drug?
- What is it for?
- How effective is it?
- How safe is it?
- Who should not receive it?
- How cost effective is it?

Your responsibility as a prescriber

- Maintain an independent stance to avoid accusations of inappropriate partiality to particular products being made.
- Adhere to the NMC Code of professional conduct[2]

---

1 The Association of the British Pharmaceutical Industry (2006). *The Code of Practice for the Pharmaceutical Industry 2006.* ABPI, London.
2 The Nursing and Midwifery Council (2004). *NMC Code of Professional Conduct: Standards for Conduct, Performance and Ethics.* (First published 08/12/2004.) NMC, London.

Hospitality and gratuities
- Get to know your local policy with regard to accepting gratuities
- Free gifts from representatives should be worth no more than £5[2]
- Be wary of offers to fund conferences etc

Useful website: 🖳 www.nofreelunch.org

Audit

An audit is a systematic and official examination of a record, process, structure, environment, or account to evaluate performance.[1]

Clinical audit

Definition

Clinical audit is conducted by doctors (medical audit) and other health care professionals (nurses, physiotherapists, occupational therapists, speech therapists, etc.) and is the systematic critical analysis of the quality of clinical caré.

Main characteristics of a clinical audit

Characteristic	Application
Topic area	Is it:
	• Relevant to the local situation?
	• Relevant to patient care?
Purpose	• Evaluation of care delivery
	• Monitoring
	• Better patient care
	• Effective use of resources
Time scale	• Short for quick results and feedback
	• Longer for a more in-depth study
Methodology	• Measurement against implicit or explicit standards
	• Opportunistic: makes use of existing data, e.g. patient's notes for a retrospective study
Feedback and dissemination	• Local (other professions, managers, purchasers, etc.)
	• National/international (conferences,
	• professional bodies, etc.)
Mechanisms of feedback and dissemination	• Internal reports
	• Audit meetings
	• Publications

---

1 Marquis, B. L,. Huston, C. J. (2000). *Leadership Roles and management Functions in Nursing* (3rd edn). Lippincot, Phialdelphia.[1]

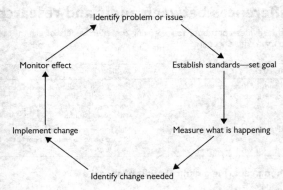

Fig. 14.1 Clinical audit cycle

2 Humphris, J. and Green, J. (2002). *Nurse prescribing*, (2nd edn). Palgrave, Basingstoke, Hampshire.

Differences between audit and research

Both activities contribute to improving the effectiveness of clinical care. The main differences are:[1]

Research	Audit
Defines or helps to define what makes up good practice.	Measures if good practice–defined by research and/or expert opinion–is being followed every day with every patient.
Advances knowledge of good practice	Helps to improve the actual quality of care being given to patients at a local level

When preparing a clinical audit proposal

Consider:
- What do you want the audit to be about?
- What do you want to achieve?
- How can the audit contribute to quality of care?
- How will you measure practice?
- How will you collect data?
- How will you get support for the audit?
- Who will support you?
- Discuss any financial assistance/funding available with the clinical effectiveness or audit department of your Trust.
- Arrange for Audit to be included in your department/directorates service plan for the next year.

(Adapted from NHS[2].)

Useful resources

National Clinical Audit Support Programme (NCASP)
   ⌨ www.nhsia.nhs.uk/phsmi/pages/ncasp.asp
Clinical Resource Audit Group (CRAG) Scotland
   ⌨ www.show.scot.nhs.uk/crag
Clinical Standards Board for Scotland (CSBS)
   ⌨ www.clinicalstandards.org
Health of Wales (HOWIS) ⌨ www.wales.nhs.uk

1 Bowling, A. (2003). *Research methods in health: investigating health and health services* (2nd ed). Open University Press, Buckingham.
2 NHS Executive (2000). *Achieving effective practice. a clinical effectiveness and research information pack for nurses, midwives and health visitors. No. 6: Preparing a proposal for clinical audit.* Stationary Office, London.

Prescription analysis and cost tabulation (PACT)

Since 1988, the introduction of computerized prescribing information at the Prescription Pricing Authority (PPA)[1] has enabled prescription analysis and costing reports to be made available to Trusts and individual prescribers.

A wealth of prescribing information is available throughout the organizations at all levels: individual GPs, practice, PCT, RHA, and nationally.

Variations between prescribing practice can be analysed in detail, trends identified, and comparisons made.

PACT summarizes drugs and appliances prescribed over the previous 3 months. Cost comparisons are shown both locally and nationally, and an attempt is made to create an average and remove demographic discrepancies by the use of prescribing units (PUs) and ASTRO-PUs.

Prescribed items may be ascribed to:
- The patient (this is 1 for 1).
- The prescribing unit (weighted depending on patient types, i.e. a surgery with a predominance of older patients is expected to prescribe more items per head than a surgery where the catchment area is a university, here the predominance will be younger patients who, it is expected, will be healthier and require fewer prescriptions).
- ASTRO-PU (adjusted for age, sex, temporary resident originated prescribing unit)
- STAR-PU (adjusted for specific therapeutic group, age–sex related prescribing units).

Further reading

Chaplin, S. (1998). National and regional prescribing trends in England. *Prescriber* 19 (January) 39–42.

1 PPA (2005). Prescribing Units. Available at ⊞ www.ppa.org.uk/ppa/info_sys/info_sys_ePACTnet _CT.htm (accessed 27 August 2005).

Cost effective prescribing

At the inception of nurse prescribing prescriptions cost the NHS £18 million every day.[1] Costs have continued to rise and the PPA recorded between 2003/04 a rise in volume of prescriptions of 5.8% and a rise in costs of 8.6%[2] and a cost of Community prescribing alone of £8.080 million.[3]

It is therefore the responsibility of the NP to always consider the cost of any items prescribed as it is essential to optimize the total NHS budget and avoid waste of resources.

Remember the *Consider the product of choice* acronym, **EASE**[4]:

E – how EFFECTIVE is the product?
A – is it APPROPRIATE for this patient?
S – how SAFE is it?
E – is the prescription cost EFFECTIVE?

- Consider recommending an OTC product which often costs the patient less than a prescription and costs the NHS nothing.
- Prescribe a drug by the generic name.
- Nurses must always use the generic name when prescribing except in the case of dressings or appliances ('the exception is where bioavailability problems are so important that the patient should always receive the same brand; in such cases, the brand name or the manufacturer should be stated.' (BNF)[5].

NB: the above now also pertains to nurses when prescribing as supplementary prescribers.

Information regarding the relative costs of prescribable items may be obtained for the Drug Tariff published on behalf of the Department of Health by The Stationery Office.

📖 Over the counter drugs (OTCs).
📖 Safe prescribing.

Further reading

🖥 www.dh.gov.uk/PublicationsAnd/Statistics

1 Prescription prescribing Authority (1996). *Annual report April 1996 to March 1997*. PPA, Newcastle on Tyne.
2 Prescription prescribing Authority (2004). *Annual report April 2003 to March 2004*. PPA, Newcastle on Tyne.
3 Department of Health (2004). *Cost of prescribing for the Community*. Health and Social care Information Centre, London.
4 Nurse Prescribing Bulletin (1999). Vol 1 No 1. NPC, Liverpool.
5 Royal Pharmaceutical Society of Great Britain (1997). *From Compliance to Concordance. Achieving shared goals in medicine taking*. RPS, London.

Evidence-based prescribing

What is evidence-based prescribing (EBP)?

Evidence-based prescribing involves the application of rigorous methodology to support the assessing of all available evidence to facilitate a safe, effective, and cost-effective prescribing decision in order to deliver the best treatment and care available. In order to further best practice it is important to disseminate the findings of audit and research. Evidence of your prescribing practice can be referred to in your appraisal and key knowledge and skills which you need to acquire can be identified to further your career and to advance best practice.

The benefits of EBP
- Improves clinical practice
- Improves outcome for patients
- Highlights the use of less effective prescribing practices.

Evidence-based prescribing decisions must be based on rigorous considerations about the efficacy of the treatment and of its clinical effectiveness.

Points to consider when evaluating the evidence
- What is the best available evidence?
- How will it effect/change existing evidence-based practice?
- What will be the health outcomes for the patient?
- Clinical and cost effectiveness
- Disseminating information.

Good sources of evidence
- BNF
- Bulletins MeReC, Bandolier etc.
- The National Prescribing Centre
- Medicines.org
- Journals (e.g. Clinical Evidence)
- Medicines' Compendium
- The Association of the British Pharmaceutical Industry (ABPI)
- National Institute of Health and Clinical Excellence (NICE).

Sources of data
- Systematic reviews and data bases for example the Cochrane library and database
- Local prescribing support services/Pharmaceutical advisor
- PACT/ EPACT (local and national prescribing audit)
- Drug bulletins/information service
- The National Prescribing Centre (NPC)
- Cochrane Database, Centre for Reviews and Dissemination
- Locally provided education/training
- Locally/regionally developed guidelines/information/research/case studies
- Support networks
- The Committee for Safety on Medicines (CSM)
- The National Health Service Executive.

Examples of some guidelines and protocols
- jointly developed locally between, nurses, GPs, pharmacists and AHP prescribers e.g. local formularies based on national evidence and best practice
- prodigy in primary care evidence?
- NICE technical appraisals

Best practice

Best practice is:
- up-to-date
- benchmarked against comparative sources where available
- in line with to local and national guidelines.

Prescribing practice analysis (audit) suggested good practice
- Suggested breakdown of data by therapeutic area.
- Review of PACT data (recommended quarterly).
- Prescription pricing authority (PPA) reviews provide potential for savings by prescribing generic medicines.
- Benchmarking against other areas and other prescribers is best practice.

PACT data

PACT data in primary care can be used to:
- review prescribing habits
- monitor adherence to prescribing policies
- compare performance between prescribers
- monitor expenditure and cost-effectiveness.

Prescribing data is monitored locally in secondary care.

Local and national formulary development and maintenance

Provides: rational, evidence based policies.
Considers: cost in context of appropriate care.
Needs: regular updating and maintenance.

Sources which support clinical appraisal skills
- Critical Appraisal Skills Programme
- Centre for Evidence Based Medicine
- Centre for Evidence Based Nursing
- National Prescribing Centre
- Nurse Prescriber web site
- Patient medication records

Inductive and deductive reasoning

Analysis of evidence is based on:
- deductive reasoning (if a and b are true, then c will follow)
- inductive reasoning (based on likelihood of probability rather than certainty)
- arguments from authority (based on accurately reported reasoning from a respected authority.

Evaluating the evidence

When evaluating the evidence from drug companies ask:
- How biased are the claims about evidence?
- How do you know the level of bias or accurate reporting?
- Would you prescribe any of these products?
- Why should you prescribe this drug?
- Why shouldn't you prescribe this drug?
- How did you come to your decision?
- How did the evidence rank in the hierarchy of evidence?
- Who sponsors the trials?
- What is the methodology?
- How many subjects were in the cohort (pre and post marketing)?
- How old were the subjects?
  See chapter on working with the drug industry

Methods of researching evidence are ranked according to their quality and their credibility.[1]

1 Granby, T. (2005). Evidence Based Prescribing. *Nurse Prescriber*, **2**(2). (21/02/05). Cited in: www.nurse-prescriber.co.uk/Articles/Evidence-based_Px.htm
2 Jones, C. (2002). Research Methods. *Pharmaceutical Journal* **28**, 839–42.

Table 15.1 To illustrate hierarchy of evidence in relation to prescribing. Adapted from Jones[2]

Rank number	Type of evidence	What is it?	Comments
Number 1	Systematic reviews	Published and unpublished research is collated and each piece is assessed by independent reviewer The results are then combined and findings discussed	(Gold standard) The most rigorous form of research
Number 2. Randomized control trials.	Used to assess relative effects of a treatment by comparing a group who are being treated with the new drug to an identical a group who are identical in every way other than that they are not being treated (the control group)		Ranked along with systematic reviews as the gold standard
Cohort studies	Observational studies of those who are being treated with a new drug	Subjects may be followed up over a long time period	
Case control studies	A group of patients who are for example taking the drug in question are studied for their medical histories which are compared to other patients within the group to look for similarities and for emergent patterns	Faster production of results than cohort studies but not as reliable	
Cross sectional surveys	Used to measure the frequency of risk factors in patients who are for example taking a drug within a defined population and a particular time		
Case reports and case studies	Descriptions of medical histories of single patients. This is then compared to case histories of patients how have similar case reports. This can be useful when searching for rarer side effects.	Not valid statistically because lacking a comparative control group	

Qualitative evidence

Remember that it is also of utmost importance to consider evidence relating to participants lived experiences (qualitative evidence) as these reflect quality of life issues which may affect concordance.

When reading a paper

Consider the potential risk and benefits to the patient in relation to the following.

- The absolute risk to the patient—e.g. how does taking the new drug reduce the patient's risk of dying?
- The absolute risk reduction. By what percentage as measured against the control group (those who have not taken the drug) can taking the new drug reduce the patient's risk of dying?
- The relative risk—e.g. what are the chances of the patients dying from the condition which is being treated if they do not have the drug in relation to the population in general?
- Relative risk reduction—how much the risk of dying from the condition which is being treated is reduced in the group who are taking the drug in comparison to the percentage risk of dying as a result of the condition for members of the control group (those who have been selected for the trial but who have not taken the drug)?
- Numbers needed to treat—how many patients will need to be treated before the effects of the new drug become evident?
- Odds ratio—how effective is the drug in comparison to it not being effective? The number of times that a treatment is effective is divided by the number of times it is not effective (any number greater than one indicates a good odds ratio).

Managing the role

Clinical supervision

Definition

[A] term used to describe a formal process of professional support and learning which enables practitioners to develop knowledge and competence, assume responsibility for their own practice and enhance consumer protection and safety of care in complex situations.

Central to the process of learning and to the expansion of scope of practice clinical supervision should be seen as a means of encouraging self assessment and analytical and reflective skills." Department of Health[1] (our italics).

Aims

- The development of professional expertise.
- The development of quality care.
- A safeguard for standards of practice
- Issues from clinical supervision will feed into the more strategic clinical governance arena.

Components

- **Educational:** development of the skills, attitudes, understanding, and abilities of an individual practitioner.
- **Restorative:** provision of an emotionally supportive environment to allow and help practioners to explore their feeling regarding their therapeutic work with patients and clients.
- **Managerial:** provision of an opportunity for quality control and a consideration of the organizational responsibilities of the individual.

Action for the supervisor

- Confirm a common belief and purpose for clinical supervision possibly through use of a contract (see below).
- Commit energy and time to the role of supervisor.
- Listen to the individual and be led by their agenda and style for learning.
- Identify how a practitioner can learn from both the positive and negative influences of practice.
- Be confident and explore new ideas, providing support as well as challenge.
- Promise respect, mutual trust, confidentiality, and sensitivity.

Example of the components of a clinical supervision contract

Contract must be clear and agreed by all
- Statement of the purpose of supervision (see above).
- Focus of supervision, i.e. reflection by the supervisees.
- An explicit statement of the responsibilities of the supervisor/ supervisee or group.
- Venue.
- Time, frequency, and length of each session.

1 Deparment of Health (1993). A vision for the future. Report of the Chief Nursing Officer. DoH, London.

- Respect for confidentiality.
- How could best practice identified in other areas be modified to suit local conditions?
- Note taking, i.e. type of notes and an agreement that secretarial support will include typing the notes of meetings.
- Evaluation of each session.
- Dates set to review points that require action.
- Signatures of the parties and date.

NB: it is important to include a mutually agreed plan of action regarding what to do if a breach of the NMC Code of Conduct is identified.

📖 NMC Code of Professional Conduct.

Remember

- Clinical supervisions meetings are not a confessional.
- Ensure time for support and identification of developmental needs.
- It can only be as useful as the participants want it to be.
- Group work may be helpful for reflection on practice.

Clinical supervision at the local level, results in clinical effectiveness for the organization and patient, which in turn leads into the more strategic arena of clinical governance.

📖 Reflection.

Further reading and help for clinical supervision

Butterworth. T., Carson, J., White, E, et al. (1997). *It is good to talk:. An evaluation study of clinical supervision in 23 sites in England and Scotland.* University of Manchester, Manchester.

RCN (2002). Lesson cards "invaluable assistance" to clinical governance. Quality Improvement Network news. Winter 2002/03, London.

RCN Facilitator and Participant packs. Realising Clinical Effectiveness and Clinical Governance through Clinical Supervision Radcliffe Medical Press Ltd, Oxford. 🖳 http://www.sci.gov.uk

Scottish Department of Health (1997). *Designed to care.* SoDoH. 🖳 www.scotland.gov.uk/ Publications.

Clinical governance (CG)

Definition

Clinical Governance is a framework which helps all clinicians, including nurses—to continuously improve quality and safeguard standards of care[1].

Places quality at the centre of both NHS reforms and through the Care Standards Act (2000)[2] applies across the independent sector.

Aims to

- Improve the quality of information for both patients and staff.
- Promote collaboration, partnership and team working.
- Reduce variations in practice.
- Implement EBP, including the use of audit and practice development.

Adapted from the RCN key principles for CG

- Focus on improving quality care.
- Apply to all health care regardless of the venue for delivery.
- Public and patient involvement is essential.
- Demands partnership between all professional groups and patients.
- Nurses have a key role to play in the implementation of CG.
- An enabling culture is needed which celebrates success and learns from mistakes.

CG resources

Commission for Patient and Public involvement in health (CPPIH): 🖳 www.doh.gov.uk/involvingpatients

Common Services Agency (Scotland) 🖳 http://www.show.scot.nhs.uk/csa www.show.scot.nhs.uk/csa

Modernisation Agency 🖳 www.modern.nhs.uk

Clinical governance Support team (CGST) 🖳 www.cgsupport.org

Changing Workforce programme 🖳 www.modern.nhs.uk

NHS Information Authority (NHSIA): 🖳 www.nhsia.nhs.uk/phsmi/clinicalgovernance

NHS performance indicators: 🖳 www.doh.gov.uk/nhsperformanceindicators

Further reading

DoH (1997) *The New NHS: modern, dependable.* The Stationary Office. London.

RCN (2002) *Lesson cards "Invaluable assistance to clinical governance. Quality Improvement Network News".* Winter 2003/03.

1 RCN (1998). In RCN (2003) *Clinical Governance- an RCN resource Guide.* RCN. London. 🖳 www.rcn.org.uk

2 Department of Health (2000) *Care Standards Act.* The Stationary Office. London.

Table 16.1 Clinical Governance underpinning policy and support

Country	Policy/legislation	Support
England	The new NHS modern dependable (DoH 1997)	Clinical Governance Support team – established 1999 – Contact on: www.cgsupport.org 0116 295 2080
Northern Ireland	Beat practice–best care. Incorporated in: The Health and Personal Social Services (quality and Improvement and Regulation) Order (2003)	Clinical and Social Care Governance Support team Contact: www.dhsspsni.gov.uk
Scotland	Designed to Care Partnership for care	NHS Quality improvement Scotland ▣ www.clinicalstandards.org
Wales	Putting Patients First	Clinical Governance Support & development Unit

Continuous professional development (CPD)

It is vital for patient safety and the enhancement of care that nurse practitioners continuously monitor and evaluate their expertise to prescribe within their field of practice.

Nurse practitioners have a professional responsibility NMC (2004) to ensure that their practice is up to date and a shared duty, with their employer, to rectify any deficits in skills and knowledge via the Clinical Supervision and Governance pathways.

NMC Code of Conduct 6.1 states

> You must keep your knowledge and skills up-to-date throughout your working life. In particular you should take part regularly in learning activities that develop your competence and performance.[1]

The Department of Health through the Lifelong Learning Strategy provides support for both the extension of the skills and knowledge of the individual and the delegation of roles and responsibilities down the escalator where that is appropriate.

www.doh.gov.uk/hrinthehs/learning/section4b/skillsescalatorhomepage.htm

The National Prescribing Center (NPC) have produced a framework to help nurses identify their needs for CPD.[2]

Further reading

Martin, R. (1999). *Clinical governance a practical guide for primary care teams.* Department of Health, London.

Phipps, K., Bowie, C., Budd, Schiller, G. (1998). *Clinical governance from rhetoric to reality.* Department of Health, London

Internet resources

▢ www.npc.co.uk—Gives information about CPD and competence.

▢ www.druginfozone.nhs.uk—a huge amount of information on medicines, prescribing and links to other sites. Some useful presentations e.g. Adverse Drug Reactions and Pharmacokinetics.

▢ www.healthcareproductions.co.uk—offers web based CPD in nurse prescribing and eczema management, with the opportunity to study to level 3

▢ www.nurses.info/nurse_prescribing.htm

▢ www.mca.gov.uk

1 NMC (2004). *Code of conduct.* p.9 Available at: ▢ www.nmc-uk.org/codeofconduct, accessed 23.08.05.
2 NPC (2001). *Maintaining Competency in Prescribing: An outline Framework to Help Nurse Prescribers.* NPC Liverpool.

Change management

Davidhizar[1] suggests there are three main **drivers for change** in contemporary health care:
- technology
- information availability
- growing populations.

The shortage of doctors and a decrease in junior doctors' hours are additional parts of the catalyst that brought about nurse prescribing.

Marquis and Houston[2] outline feelings of loss, stress, achievement, and pride as normal reactions to change, and cite the need of a change agent to make the process successful.

Change agent

Definition

A person skilled in the theory and implementation of planned change, who possesses well-developed leadership and management skills.

Change theory was identified in the mid 1900s by Kurt Lewin,[3] who described three phases through which the process must go before a planned change becomes part of a system.

- *Unfreezing*: here the change agent persuades those opposing the change of its necessity
- *Movement*: the change agent has to ensure that the driving forces for the change exceed the restraining forces of the system. If possible, change should be approached gradually to enable those involved to be fully assimilated in the change
- *Refreezing*: to ensure that the change becomes integrated into the normal working patterns, the change agent needs to support the adaptive efforts of those adopting the change.

Change strategies

Because many change agents within nurse prescribing do not have a hierarchical power base and are attempting to influence their peers and fellow professionals, a *normative–re-educative strategy*, which uses group process, may well be appropriate:

- The change agent assumes that because humans are social animals, they are more influenced by others than by facts
- Skill with interpersonal relationships enables the change agent to focus on non-cognitive determinants of behaviour, such as roles, relationships, attitudes, and feelings.

Change resisters

Silber[4] suggests that a person's ability to cope with change rests on:
- their flexibility to events
- their evaluation of the immediate situation
- the anticipated consequences of the change
- what is in it for them, what they have to lose or gain.

1 Davidhizar, R. (1996). Surviving organizational change. *Health Care Supervisor*, **14**(4), 19–24.
2 Marquis, B.L. and Houston, C. (2000). *Leadership roles and management functions in nursing*, (3rd edn). Lippincott, Philadelphia.
3 Lewin, K. (1951). *Field theory in social sciences*. Harper & Row, New York.
4 Silber, M.B. (1993). The 'C's' in excellence: Choice and change. *Nursing Management*, **24** (9), 60–2.

Section 5

Responsibilities

Responsibilities

Where to get up-to-date information

National guidelines

The National Institute for Health and Clinical Excellence (NICE), provides up to date technology appraisals. These are nationally recognized guidelines which adhere to the best clinical evidence base and account for best practice and cost effective prescribing. Technology appraisals are updated every five years.

Nationally recognized guidelines are also produced by:
- The British Thoracic society (BTS) ⌨ www.brit.thoracic.org.uk
- The British Hypertensive Society (BHS) ⌨ www.bhs.org.uk
- The British Diabetic Association (BDA) ⌨ www.diabetes.org.uk
- The British Heart Foundation (BHF) ⌨ www.bhft.org.uk
- The Scottish Intercollegiate Guidelines Network (SIGN)
  ⌨ www.sign.ac.uk

Prodigy, ⌨ www.prodigy.nhs.uk, provides a nationally recognized knowledge source for extended and supplementary prescribers in primary and secondary care.

Local guidelines

Guidelines exist to help direct the prescriber to the best, safest and most effective evidence-based prescribing. Guidelines do not seek to impose and, in supplementary prescribing, in agreement with the doctor independent prescriber and the patient, can be tailored to meet the needs of the individual patient. However, whenever possible, it is best practice for the nurse prescriber working for the National Health Service (NHS) to follow the guidelines as indicated both nationally and, if working in the NHS, within the local NHS formulary.

Locally-produced NHS formularies provide evidence-based guidelines, formularies and protocols for prescribing medications and appliances, which also recommend for locally-accepted practice, safe and cost effective prescribing.

PACT data

PACT and SPA (Scottish Prescribing Analysis) are available as audit reports of practitioners prescribing on a quarterly (three-monthly) basis. This data provides comparison between local and national prescribing patterns and can be broken down to indicate individual prescribing patterns. (📖 Reflective practice.)

The Drug Tariff

The Drug Tariff is produced monthly as a joint compilation between the Department of Health and the Prescription Pricing Authority.[1] Now known as the NHS Business Services Authority.

Useful information contained in the Drug Tariff includes:
- The basic price of named drugs, appliances and chemical reagents.
- Endorsements including pack sizes.
- Whether the prescription is in pharmacopoeial or generic form.
- Brand name and name of manufacturer or wholesaler from whom the drug was purchased.
- Quantity supplied (if at variance with quantity ordered).
- Pharmacists' professional payments fees.
- Commonly used pack sizes.
- Advice on domicillary oxygen service.
- Advice to care homes.
- Borderline substances.
- The dental prescribing formulary.
- The district nurse and health visitor prescribers' formulary.
- The nurse prescribers' extended formulary.
- Drugs and other substances not to be prescribed under the NHS pharmaceutical services (blacklisted drugs).
- Drugs to be prescribed in certain circumstances under the NHS pharmaceutical services.

1 Department of Health (2005). *Drug Tariff* (latest edn). HMSO, London.

Review of prescribing web sites

🖳 http://www.pharmj.com **(The Pharmaceutical Journal)**
This is the electronic version of *The Pharmaceutical Journal*. Subscription is free and it provides an excellent source of evidence-based information including continuing professional development (CPD) with a pharmacist-based slant. The web site links to *Clinical Evidence*, BMJ publishing group. This publication has up to date reviews of clinical evidence related to prescribing. It is useful for systematic reviews of up to date randomized control trials and clinical comparisons of drugs and their applications.

🖳 www.prodigy.nhs.uk **(Prodigy)**
This site provides patient, nurse, and doctor information for a wide range of disease management. The site provides brief updates which inform practice. The site also provides information leaflets with patient friendly diagrams as well as details of self-help groups, patient groups, and similar organizations.

🖳 www.abpi.org.uk **(Association of the British Pharmaceutical Industry)**
This site contains useful information pertaining to the drug industry, their code of conduct and vital statistics. The site includes some drug company produced patient information and summaries of product characteristics.

🖳 http://www.am-publishing.co.uk/prescriber.html **(Prescriber)**
The online electronic journal *Prescriber* covers peer reviewed articles relating to primary care, therapeutics and prescribing related issues. Good for research articles about pharmacology and pharmacokinetics and dynamics. The site links to NICE guidelines and NSFs and also has medical humour.

🖳 http://www.npc.co.uk **(NPC-National Prescribing Centre)**
Contains links relating to clinical governance, knowledge and skills framework, standards and competencies related to prescribing. This site provides authoritative and up to date information on all aspects of medical and non medical prescribing. The site also produces MeReC bulletins.

🖳 http://www.mhra.gov.uk **(Medicines and Health Care Regulatory Agency)**
This excellent site is devoted to protecting the public, maintaining and regulating standards for the pharmaceutical industry and prescribing. It provides comprehensive information on how products are licensed and information related to prescribing and public health.

🖳 http://www.nelh.nhs.uk **(NeLH-National electronic Library for Health)**
Provides links to all major academic and information sites for prescribing, including BNF, Cochrane data base, *Clinical Evidence* and *Drugs and Therapeutics Bulletin*.

▣ http://www.sign.ac.uk **(SIGN-Scottish Intercollegiate Guidelines Network)**
Links with NICE, to work in partnership to provide evidence-based guidelines for standardized treatment for disease management. This site is the Scottish equivalent of NICE. Good reliable source of evidence-based information.

▣ http://www.ukmi.nhs.uk **(UKMIPG-UK Medicines Information Pharmacists Group)**
This site is a source of up-to-date online information for pharmacists working in primary care. Useful links to National electronic Library for Medicine www.nlm.nih.gov/databases and specialist advice services. Interesting link to www.quackwatch.com.

▣ www.medicines.org.uk
Provides summary of product characteristics for drugs and a search engine for information regarding specific medicines.

▣ http://www.freemedicaljournals.com/index.htm
This site provides access to useful free online journals.

▣ www.dotpharmacy.com/prevwks1.html **(Chemist and Druggist)**
Useful for self-testing for CPD.

▣ http://www.which.net/health/dtb/main.html **(Drug and Therapeutics Bulletin)**
Up-to-date information regarding common drugs.

▣ http://www.pharmj.com/backissues.html **(Hospital Pharmacist)**
Contains lots of information about medicine management. Good access to free electronic journals related to prescribing. Useful updates from *The Pharmaceutical Journal* on line.

▣ http://www.jr2.ox.ac.uk/bandolier **(Bandolier)**
Rich source for evidence-based pharmacology and prescribing information.

▣ http://bmj.com/ **(BMJ-British Medical Journal)**
Access to evidence-based medicine, news and reviews.

▣ http://www.bnf.org/ **(British National Formulary)**
This site provides online up to date BNF if you are a subscriber. Lots of links to useful sites related to prescribing.

Regional Medicines Information Services

Regional Medicines Information Services, also known as United Kingdom Medicines Information Services (UKMi), provides, NHS pharmacist and technician advice for all health care professionals.

All Medicines information activities can be accessed on the UKMi website at: 🖳 www.ukmi.nhs.uk Links are available to other related sites such as UKMi central and Druginofzone providing region specific information.

This service provides prescribing information and advice regarding:
- pregnancy
- breast feeding
- alternative medicines
- complementary therapies
- news and e mail alerts
- bulletins
- product updates and information.

Purchasing and supplies Agency (PASA)
- Regarding alerts and drug shortages
- Patent expiry
- Changes to product characteristic summaries.

Information on new drugs
- Provides information on drugs tracked through clinical development phases 2 and 3
- Provides evaluated appraisals on drugs likely to make an impact on NHS prescribing
- Service and Financial Framework (SAFF) planning.

Support for evidence based practice
- FAQ data base
- Critical appraisal trials (CATs)
- Toolkits for the National Service frameworks (NSFs)
- Available evaluations for complementary medicines
- One stop reference shop.

Training
- UKMi workbook providing tutorials facilitating user access to information on particular aspects of prescribing.
- MiCAL: a CD-Rom which includes details of critical appraisal literature searching and information sources.
- Packages for Regional pharmacy training programmes.

Shared care guidelines
Details of prescribing committee decisions and project information.

Support for national organizations
- NHS Direct
- Walk in centers
- National Electronic Library for health (NeHL)

- National Patient Safety Agency
- Some are part of the National Poisons Information service.

Local medicines information support
- Enquiry answering service for all health professionals.
- Local bulletins
- Clinical pharmacy, Clinical Governance and Medicines management support
- Educational support.

Advice and Support
Advisory Committee on Borderline Substances
NICE
🖥 www.nice.org.uk

Action on Smoking and Health
ASH
🖥 www.ash.org

Age Concern
General enquiries: 0208 765 7200
Info. Line: 0800 009966
🖥 www.ageconcern.co.uk

Alcohol Concern
E mail: contact@alcoholcncern.org.uk
🖥 www.alcoholconcern.org.uk

Allergy UK
Telephone: 0208 303 8525
🖥 www.allergyfoundation.com

Alzheimer's Society
Telephone: 0845 300 0326
E mail: enquiries@alzheimers.org.uk
🖥 www.alzeheimers.org.uk

Anaphylaxis Campaign
Telephone: 01252 542029
E mail: Info@anaphylaxis.org.uk
🖥 www.anaphylaxis.org.uk

Asthma UK
Telephone: 0845 701 0203 (Mon-Fri 9am-5pm)
🖥 www.asthma.org.uk

Blood Pressure Association
🖥 www.bpassoc.org.uk

British Association of Dermatologists
🖳 www.bad.org.uk

British Cardiac Society
🖳 www.bcs.com

British Dermatological Nursing Group
🖳 www.bdng.org.uk

British Heart Foundation
Telephone heart information line: 0845 070 8070
🖳 www.bhf.org.uk

British Herbal Medicines Association (BHMA)
🖳 www.trusthomeopathy.org

British Kidney Patient Association (BKPA)
Telephone: 0142 047 2021/2 (9am–5pm)
🖳 www.britishkidney-pa.co.uk

British Lung Foundation
E mail: enquiries@blf-uk.org
🖳 www/lunguk.org/support-groups.asp

British Menopause Society
🖳 www.the–bms.org

British Pregnancy Advisory service (BPAS)
Actionline telephone: 0845 730 4030
🖳 www.bpas.org

British Thoracic Society
E mail: bts@brit-thoracic.org.uk
🖳 www.brit-thoracic.org.uk

British Thyroid Foundation
🖳 www.btf-thyroid.org

British Vascular Foundation
E mail: bvf@care4free.net
🖳 www.bvf.org.uk

Cancer Bacup
Helpline telephone: 0808 800 1234 (Mon- Fri. 9am–7pm)
🖳 www.cancerbacup.org.uk

Colon Cancer Concern
Infoline telephone: 0870 506 050 (Mon- Fri. 10am–4pm)
E mail: info@coloncancer.org.uk
🖳 www.coloncancer.org.uk

Colostomy Association
Telephone: Freephone helpline: 0800 587 6744
🖥 www.colostomyassociation.org.uk

The Continence Foundation
Helpline telephone: 0845 345 0165 (Mon- Fri. 9.30am–1pm)
E mail: continence-help@dialpipex.com
🖥 www.continence-foundation.org.uk

Carers Line
Telephone: 0808 808 7777 (Mon- Fri. 10am–12 and 2pm–4pm)

The Depression Alliance
🖥 www.depressionalliance.org

Diabetes UK
Careline telephone: 0845120 2960 (Mon–Fri. 9am–5pm) (lo-call rate)
E mail: info@diabetes.org.uk
🖥 www.diabetes.org.uk

The Disability Information Trust
🖥 www.abilityonline.org.uk/disability.information.trust.htm

The Disabled Living Foundation
Telephone: 0845 130 9177 (low-call rate)
Text Phone: 020 7432 8009 (Mon–Fri. 10.00am–1pm)
🖥 www.dlf.org.uk

Family Heart Association
E mail: md@familyheart.org
🖥 www.familyheart.org

The Ileostomy and Internal Pouch Support Group (ia)
Freephone: 0800 018 4724
E mail: info@the-ia.org.uk
🖥 www.the-ia.org.uk

The Impotence Association
Helpline telephone: 0870 774 3571
E mail: info@sda.uk.net
🖥 www.sda.uk.net

Irritable Bowel Syndrome (IBS) Network
Telephone: 01543 492192 (Mon–Fri. 6am–8pm, Sat 10am–12 noon)
E mail: info@ibsnetwork.org.uk
🖥 www.ibsnetwork.org.uk

Long-Term Medical Conditions Alliance (LMCA)
E mail: info@lmca.org.uk
🖳 www.lmca.org.uk

Marie Stopes International
Telephone-One call:
Abortion, emergency contraception: 0845 300 8090
Vasectomy, female sterilization: 0845 300 02 12
Health Screening: 0845 300 0460
E mail: info@mariestopes.org.uk
🖳 www.mariestopes.org.uk

The Menopause Amarant Trust
Helpline telephone: 01293 413 000 (Mon–Fri. 11.00am–6pm)
🖳 www.amarantmenopausetrust.org.uk

National Eczema Society
Helpline telephone: 0870241 3604 (Mon–Fri. 8am–8pm)
🖳 www.eczema.org

National Fertility Association (ISSUE)
Helpline telephone: 01922 722 888
E mail: info@issue.c.uk
🖳 www.infertilitynetworkuk.com

National Osteoporosis Society (NOS)
Helpline telephone: 0845 450 0230
E mail: info@nos.org.uk
🖳 www.nos.org.uk

National Prescribing Centre
Telephone: 0151 794 8134
🖳 www.npc.co.uk

National Respiratory Training Centre
Health professional helpline telephone: 01926 493 63
E mail: enquiries@nrts.org.uk
🖳 www.nrts.org.uk

Necrobiosis Support Network
Telephone: 020 7878 2308

NHS Stop Smoking Helpline
Telephone: 0800 169 0169

Nurses Hypotension Association
E mail: secretary@nha.uk.net
🖳 www.nha.uk.net

Nursing and Midwifery Council (NMC)
Telephone: 020 7637 7181
🖥 www.nmc.uk.org

The British Pain Society
E mail info@britishpainsociety.org
🖥 www.britishpainsociety.org

The Paracetamol Information Centre
E mail gb@butlers.u-net.com
🖥 www.pharmweb.net/paracetamol.htm

The Psoriasis Association
Telephone: 0845 676 0076 (Mon–Thurs. 9.15–4.45pm Fri. 9.15–4.30pm)
🖥 www.psoriasis-assocaition.org.uk

The Royal College of Nursing (RCN)
Information and advice for members- telephone: 0845 772 6100
🖥 www.rcn.org.uk

The Samaritans
Telephone: 08457 909090 (charged at local rates)
E mail Jo@samaritans.org
🖥 www.samaritans.org

Smoking Cessation Action in Primary care (SCAPE)
30 Orange Street,
London. WC2H 71Z

Urostomy Association
Telephone: 01245 224 294 (10am–12am)

Women's Health Concern
Counselling and advice- E mail: counseling@womens-health-concern.org
🖥 www.womens-health-concern.org

Wound Care Society
🖥 www.woundcaresociety.org

Additional prescribing information available in the BNF

The Community Practitioners' Formulary/British National Formulary (CPF/BNF) contains invaluable information for the nurse prescriber, both in the notes on drugs and preparations and in the various appendices.

The UK health departments distribute BNFs to NHS hospitals and prescribing doctors and nurses. It is available free online to NHS staff at: ⊞ www.bnf.org

Requests for extra copies and details of changes for mailing may be made by contacting the NHS Response line on: 08701 555 455.

Pharmaid

Even BNFs which are 6–12 months old are of use for those working in developing countries.

The Commonwealth Pharmaceutical Association has a scheme, **Pharmaid,** which despatches older BNFs, in the month of November, to areas where they may be of use.

Please contact www.pharmaid.com or check the health related press for details of this scheme.

Additional prescribing information available within appendices of the BNF

- Drug interactions.
- Liver disease.
- Renal impairment.
- Pregnancy and breastfeeding.
- Intravenous additives.
- Borderline substances.
- Wound management products and elastic hosiery.
- Cautionary and advisory labels for dispensing.
- Basic net prices (see Drug Tariff, published monthly, for information. OTCs are at retail price which includes VAT).
- Changes to the names of drugs in accordance with the EEC directive 92/27/EEC. This states that where the British Approved Name (BAN) is different from the Recommended International Non-proprietary name (rINN), the BAN must be changed to the rINN.
- Index of manufacturers and their contact details.
- Index of 'special order' manufacturers.
- A table of approximate conversions:
  - lbs and stones to kg
  - fl.oz to ml
  - Imperial to metric length
  - Mass
  - Volume
  - Other units.

- Table for ideal body weight, height, and surface area for children aged newborn–12 years, and adults, male and female.
- Contact details for:
  - The Driver and Vehicle Licensing Authority (DVLA)
  - Medications prohibited for sportsmen and women
  - Poisons information services
  - Travel immunisation requirements
  - Patient information lines
  - Medicines information services.

Working outside the UK

Working outside the UK

The requirements, registration, permits, and qualifications vary from country to country within the European Union (EU) and from state to state within other countries. It is therefore advisable to check the specifics with each embassy. General advice follows regarding:

- Australia
- USA
- working within the European Union (EU).

Australia

To practice as a registered nurse in Australia you need to follow the procedure outlined below.

- Be registered as a nurse by the board of the state/territory in which you wish to practice.
- You will also need to have already applied for and received the relevant visa/work permit entitling you to work.
- Each state or territory has its own legislation and arrangements regarding nurses from overseas.
- If you are not registered you cannot work. One of the easiest and cheapest states in which to register is New South Wales (NSW).

Registration

- The Australian Nursing Council Incorporated (ANCI) Assessment is a requirement before initial registration is possible.
- Application forms and detailed information is available on their web site.
- Once registered in one state it is relatively easy to transfer your registration to another state.

Visas and work permits

Categories

If you are a citizen of the UK, Republic of Ireland, Canada, or the Netherlands, and/or if you are aged between 18 and 25 years or between 26 and 30 years at the time of application and can show your entry to Australia will be of benefit to both yourself and Australia you are eligible for a working holiday visa (WHV).

To obtain a WHV

- You need to apply to the Australian High Commission before you leave.
- It is illegal to enter Australia without your WHV.
- This type of visa allows you to work for up to 3 months with one employer and for a total of 12 months.

If you do not fall into the categories listed above you will need a work permit (WP).

To obtain a WP

- Firstly you need to be offered a position or be sponsored by someone to work.
- A WP allows you to work for over 3 months and up to 4 years.

Useful contact addresses
Australian High Commission,
Migration branch,
Strand,
London WC2B 4LA
▢ www.australia.org.uk

Information and application forms can be obtained from the
Department of Immigration and Multicultural and Indigenous Affairs
(DIMIA) website:
▢ www.immi.gov.au
▢ http://www.anc.org.au/registrationboards

The United States of America (USA)

In order to practice as a registered nurse in the USA you will need both a licence to practice there and a work permit.

- Salaries, conditions, and the cost of living vary from state to state and there are no national agreements.
- A car may be essential to enable you to work in some areas as hospitals are built on the outer fringes of cities.
- Annual leave entitlement may be as little as 2–4 weeks per year.
- Check your employment package includes health insurance.

In the USA there is only one category of first-level nurse; the Registered Nurse (RN). The RN qualification is the equivalent to the UK's Registered General Nurse (RGN). Only a RGN is eligible to apply for nurse registration in the USA.

Requirements

There are three main requirements for gaining employment:

- sitting and passing The Commission on Graduates of Foreign Nursing Schools (CGFNS) examination.
- once you have passed your CGFNS exam you are eligible to take the NCLEX-RN® exam in a chosen state. Joining a recruitment agency which sponsors nurses to fly to the USA is a good way of sitting and gaining this qualification.
- only New York and Florida do not require you to pass your CGFNS before you take the state exam the NCLEX-RN.

Each state has its own board of nursing and different eligibility criteria for foreign nurses.

Visa/work permits

- Prospective employers have to prove they have made every effort to recruit a person who already has the right to work and reside in the USA before they can employ foreign nurses.
- Unless you are a US citizen by marriage or by birth you must have the correct visa to enter America.
- If you work on a visitor's visa you run the risk of being deported.

For further information on gaining an employment visa and other useful immigration checks visit:
US State Department website 🖳 http://www.state.gov
National Immigration services 🖳 www.myvisa.com

The European Union (EU)

There has been some harmonization to enable movement between EU member countries and a good source of information is found at:
🖥 http://www.dfes.gov.uk/europeopen/uktoeu

Additional information on nursing abroad is obtainable for Royal College of Nursing Members at:
🖥 www.rcn.org.uk
🖥 international.office@rcn.org.uk

For independent information and a chance to contact nurses who have already experienced working abroad try:
🖥 www.21centurynurse.com

Provided you keep your up your registration you will not require a Return to Practice (RTP) course on return to working for the NHS in the UK

Index

REFERENCE